TRAPPED IN THE WEB:
HOW I LIBERATED MYSELF FROM INTERNET ADDICTION, AND HOW YOU CAN TOO

BY
A.N. TURNER
WITH BEN BEARD

Copyright © 2018 by A.N. Turner

All rights reserved. This book or any portion thereof may not be reproduced or utilized in any form or by any means without written permission by the author and publisher.

Published in the United States of America

ISBN: 978-1-7321821-9-6

Phanarion II, 2018

A.N. Turner
www.breakingthefeedbackloop.com

Design by Jamie Trubowitsch and Kris Kozak

The truth is always an abyss. One must—as in a swimming pool—dare to dive from the quivering springboard of trivial everyday experience and sink into the depths, in order to later rise again—laughing and fighting for breath—to the now doubly illuminated surface of things.

— Franz Kafka

I would like to dedicate this to the young adults of my generation who have borne the costs of the recent advance in technology—the paradigm shift of instantly accessible social and sexual entertainment. They are victims of a social experiment gone wildly awry.

TRAPPED IN THE WEB

INTRODUCTION: YOU, ME, AND EVERYONE WE KNOW

We are drowning in a sea of free information. The Internet is in our businesses and homes, our bedrooms. An army of designers and data-crunchers spend their working lives figuring out ways to make us stay plugged in longer. Our desires are being repackaged by giant tech companies and then sold back to us under the guise of free content. It isn't free. We are paying for it with intangible currencies that people are only now beginning to understand—our time, our privacy, our willpower, our relationships, and our futures.

Most ancient cultures have stories of mythological monsters of endless appetite—giant creatures that exist to devour and eat. They have no souls, no thoughts; they are nothing but gaping mouths and an infinite capacity for consumption. In *The Odyssey*, this creature is called Scylla. In 2018, it's called the Internet. It's everywhere. It's the first thing we check when we wake up, and it's the last thing we look at before we go to sleep. We are feeding the beast all day, every day.

You must change your life, Rilke said to the young poet. We must heed his advice. We have to understand the world we live in and how our relationships are being shaped by the digital age in order to change our lives, in order to find happiness. Through some simple and not so simple behavioral changes, I believe we can become more useful, more productive, and more independent. We can be truly happy.

By reshaping our relationship with the digital world, we can become torches, burning with life.

I don't profess to be able to help everyone correct

their digital relationships. Some people may need help beyond what can be found in a book. I encourage all young adults to consider how to improve their digital relationships in ways that will work for them, given the idiosyncrasies of their lives and their ingrained behaviors. For the vast majority of us, I believe that implementing the frameworks and strategies outlined in this book will result in a profound change in not only our digital relationships but also our lives.

Through research and autobiography, I explore two central questions: how are new digital technologies reducing productivity? And how can we reshape our digital relationships so we can improve ourselves, not only to find personal happiness but also for the betterment of society at large?

I have made a lot of large, sweeping generalizations that are directed specifically toward the audience for this book: ambitious young adults who have been negatively impacted by the Internet. We've allowed an amorphous mass of interconnected computers to invade our most treasured of intimacies—our personal relationships. We are a miserable generation so far, and if we don't fundamentally alter the way we interact with new technologies, we are doomed.

TRAPPED IN THE WEB

NULL-O

This book stems from a series of important realizations I had during my junior year of college at the University of Pennsylvania.

It began with a junior year internship application. I was somehow accepted into a prestigious program at a partner of Facebook, an internship with a product manager. It was a serious, real-world job with real responsibilities, and leading up to it I was nearly paralyzed with fear. I felt sick, weak, and incapable. I was too distracted. I knew I had to be more productive, but I didn't know how. I sensed the impending demands of the internship as a vise around my neck. I knew that if I didn't change my life, I wouldn't succeed. I would fail to meet the challenge of the internship, and I would fail to meet the challenge of the looming demands of the real world beyond it. I was too busy. But with what? I constantly obsessed over what other people—many of them complete strangers—were posting on Facebook, Instagram, Snapchat, or my fraternity group chat. My time was being eroded by a hundred little distractions every day. I was literally clicking my life away. I realized something else—I was depleting my sexual energy in a downward spiral of online porn consumption. I was investing my sexual passions and fantasies into digitized non-companionship. I was desensitized, enervated, lonely, weary, and way too young to feel all those things at the same time.

Aldous Huxley wrote about the future in his dystopian novel *Brave New World*. It's an eerie, disturbing read. He presents a society that hums along

A.T.

without any thought to its past or to the future. The astonishing power of the human imagination has gone terribly wrong. People ingest an astonishing array of drugs, attend sex parties, genetically modify future generations, and shuffle about in a malcontented haze. No one is happy. No one is ambitious. Nothing is accomplished. All that's left is pleasure and distraction.

I was living in Huxley's future. I couldn't concentrate. I craved instant gratification. I had terrible habits. I carried around a nagging guilt. A deep sickness and anxiety. Despite being at an Ivy League school, I felt I wasn't maturing. I wasn't getting smarter, wiser, more capable, more outgoing, more socially competent. I felt my intelligence was weakening, slipping into a morass I couldn't understand. My thinking was fragmented. I couldn't write logically. All the work that had gone into my education was not resulting in any growth. I wasn't flourishing. I felt soul-sick.

I lived on my computer. I didn't take my learning seriously. Rather, I had lost the ability to do so. I continually crammed information for quizzes and tests into my head and then dumped that information, emptying the cache in my localized server. With my increasingly digital lifestyle, I continually spent less and less time reflecting, less and less time reading. I gobbled up more and more artificial stimulation. I gorged on social media, pornography, click bait articles, TV shows, and movies. Over time, my attention span shrank and weakened; I had the cognitive attention capabilities of a young child. I was overloaded with information but hollowed out inside. I lived in a constant state of over-stimulation. I had few mental resources available. I couldn't engage with lectures, books, or papers that needed to be written. I felt underwhelmed by reality. I pursued distractions at the expense of my own development. I couldn't engage with singular tasks for sustained periods of time.

I had a compulsion to constantly consume new artificial stimulants. I was addicted.

I was a low-level social parasite, protected by privilege and giving nothing back to anyone. I was skirting by.

And almost everyone I interviewed was in the exact same situation, trapped in a matrix of our own devising. We were caught in the monster's mouth.

Almost everyone I interviewed consumed epic amounts of online pornography. These young adults and I were caught in the grip of a very subtle trap—leaching our sexual energies, destroying our motivation and desires, leaving behind lethargic creatures who had nullified the very forces that make living things so dynamic. Our romantic relationships were, almost to a person, mixed up and decidedly unromantic. We oscillated between the prurient and the pointless. We had difficulty motivating to do anything. We all did the minimum amount of work to scrape by, saving our energies for our online selves. Our avatars had richer lives than we did. Sex, lust, love, desire, video clips, images, aggregators—it was all a jumble of masturbatory sessions that, in retrospect, were grim.

Everyone was suffocating.

I wanted love, acceptance, passion, purpose. I wanted to escape the digitized fleshly fantasia that haunted my waking thoughts and bedeviled my dreams.

A.T.

My behavior with digital media and the consequences of that behavior were simply not compatible with the life I wanted to live. Society had given me a lot. I needed to live a better life. I thought if I could find a solution for myself, perhaps it could help others who were suffering from the same digital malaise.

This book is the result of my experiments.

This isn't a book about pornography. Others have written about the pornification of America, where porn concepts and memes and images have invaded our public sphere. Others have written about the vast and lucrative business of porn, the exploitation of many of its workers, and its takeover by the giant tech aggregators. This isn't a screed against pornography, either. This is a book about the consequences of consuming pornography. And those consequences are vast. A whole generation has been damaged by unfettered access to addictive pornography.

TRAPPED IN THE WEB

THE FORTRESS OF SOLITUDE

In ancient times people sought out silent contemplation in pursuit of wisdom. They believed the divine only communicated in silence. Were they so wrong? When's the last time you lived in a memory, a good one, and really explored it? Think about the best meal you ever had. Close your eyes. Envision your surroundings—a restaurant, your grandmother's kitchen, a soft patch of grass in a park on a sunny day. Recreate the sounds, the smells, the taste of the food in your mouth. Try to remember the conversation. It's beautiful, right? And it only cost you a minute or two.

Solitude combats mental overload and enables us to process information. You don't have to practice seated meditation to gain those benefits. In Proust and the Squid, author Maryanne Wolf makes the case that reading frees up parts of the mind to rest, process, and even grapple with other things. Reading, she argues, has a serious and important survival function. We need it.

Pursuing silence, quiet, contemplation, hell, even reading a book—in 2018, these sound like revolutionary acts. And in a sense, they are. By reclaiming our personal and private thoughts, we reclaim our inner lives from the Scylla of the digital age.

The titans of tech understand this too well. Satya Nadella, the CEO of Microsoft, writes: "We are moving from a world where computing power was scarce to a place where it now is almost limitless, and where the true scarce commodity is increasingly human attention." The Internet feeds on our clicks, our likes, our friends, our followers. The more we consume, the more it consumes us.

Herbert Simon, Nobel Prize winner in economics, said it best: "What information consumes is the attention of its recipients. Hence a wealth of information creates a poverty of attention." We aren't experiencing a wealth of information, but a torrential flood. And since our future currency is our attention span, we must find a way to higher ground, to a place where our most valuable resource is our own, or we will drown.

When I received my internship offer, I worried that I had become so accustomed to bad habits that no matter how determined and motivated I was to contribute during my summer internship, I would fail. I had no self-confidence, no internal reservoirs to fall back on. I didn't know how to apply myself for any stretch of time or motivate myself to do things that weren't required.

But I surprised myself. During the internship, I was able to correct my bad habits and separate from a lifestyle of continuous multitasking. I trained myself to engage in single-tasking for sustained periods of time. I sought out decompression and solitude. I craved silence and introspection. The benefit was tremendous and immediate. Whereas the summer before I had barely survived in an informal internship—an extremely casual role that should have been relatively effortless—during the more serious internship at the Facebook partner, I thrived.

I took initiative. I used some tools to create a product for visualizing customer data, which was shown to the CEO. After I presented the data visualization tool to the company, a senior engineering manager pulled me

—an intern!—into a room with his team of engineers to conduct an exploration into how that product could be spun out and sold to other companies and turned into a business.

By changing my habits, I changed my life. By changing my life, I impacted others. I didn't skulk, or hide, or leach, or pretend. I didn't skate by. I contributed. I created. I was successful.

And it felt fucking great.

A.T.

THIS IS A SELF-HELP BOOK

I want you to feel great, too.

Self-help books focus on productivity, but few of those books grapple with how to improve the underlying conditions of our work. Many gurus simply tell people to increase discipline and creativity by working harder and longer. But the reality is that most people in competitive environments are already working at their maximum discipline and creativity within the current paradigm. Most people must make changes to the underlying conditions of life in the digital age, or significant changes in their productivity, creativity, and work and life satisfaction won't ever occur. Imagine being lost, at night, in an immense primeval forest. You are surrounded by ancient trees that blot out the moonlight, jagged rocks and thorny underbrush all around, and you cannot see a thing. Working harder won't get you out of that forest. You need illumination. And a map.

And it's with this map that things get interesting. Discovering that when it comes to the forest of infinite distraction and stimulation that is the Internet, there aren't many good maps available, I decided to create one of my own. I observed and analyzed my relationship with digital media and the consequences of that relationship. I worked on devising a program.

There was trial and error. I suffered through setbacks and side alleys. I wandered. I reflected. I studied. It was inefficient, often circular, often frustrating. But I found a way out of the forest, and I want to share my map with others.

TRAPPED IN THE WEB

THE GORDIAN KNOT

I have just scratched the surface. The collective human imagination is the most potent thing in the universe. In just a few thousand years we went from living in thatch huts to establishing a permanent space station and building self-replicating machines. Now more than ever before we all have the ability to create and accomplish so much because we have instantaneous access to information and communication. We are living in the future. But here in the future we face a Gordian knot of interlocking problems: immense global suffering now, planet-wide extinction looming. Yet we squander our energies and ambitions, the very things we need to solve these problems.

What should we do? Break the Internet? Return to some impossible, Edenic, off-the-grid utopia? I'm not suggesting anything so radical. Instead, I want you to trade short-term stimulation for long-term happiness. I want you to wake up in the real world.

Change your life. Change your relationship to the Internet. You will find time, energy, purpose. You will be able to interact with people in person. You will feel more alive.

That mythical beast that only wants to eat? It turns out there is a way to defeat it. Don't feed it.

A.T.

NO TIME LIKE THE PRESENT

This is a rallying cry. We are in a time crunch.

Social norms have changed. New technologies—the cotton gin, the automobile, the airplane—always alter human civilization, and not always for the better. Yes, some of the more deleterious effects of the Internet will probably flatten out over time, but by then our youth, maybe even our lives, will have been squandered.

Young people are supposed to be taking control of their lives with unfettered access to information, but the opposite is happening. Digital media is preventing us from finding meaning or purpose. We are falling into a new age of alienation—from our work, from other people, from our very bodies. We've already witnessed the amoral, click-obsessed social networks and news aggregators hijacking our presidential election. With similarly dire consequences, millions of young people's essential selves are being hijacked by this conscience-less machine.

And it is getting worse. The potency of the distractions—when complex algorithms dictate the content in your news feed, personalized content that is, once you see it, nigh impossible to avoid clicking on—make them severely habit-forming. In fact, entire industries are popping up, attempting to monetize the cracks in our resolve. New, increasingly immersive platform technologies like virtual reality and augmented reality are emerging. New temptations. New distractions.

Coders, thinkers, and designers have access to user data and ingenious ways of mining it. They have algorithms that reveal our urges, secrets, desires, political leanings, buying habits, reading habits, listening habits, watching habits. They know things about us we often don't know about ourselves. The Internet is compromised. It exists to capture human attention, warp it, contain it, and then transmogrify it into profits. These methods of data extraction are only getting more and more canny and effective. As companies behind various forms of digital entertainment receive more data on user behavior, they are able to optimize their services to make them more psychologically appealing, reducing barriers to allow near limitless use.

We have to retool our relationships to machines. We have to exercise self-control now. It may sound like science fiction, but we risk an entire generation being subjugated by inescapable addiction. We risk Aldous Huxley's nightmarish vision, where everything is permitted, pleasure is the only pursuit, sex is loveless, and temporary derangement is the major form of recreation. We are already living in a dystopian future; a brave new world is right around the corner.

Limiting our exposure is challenging. Resisting temptation drains energy. Willpower is a finite resource. And resisting something that appears to be pleasurable feels odd, old-fashioned. Deny yourself? Why?

A.T.

WE ALL HAVE THE VIRUS

The Walking Dead posits a contemporary America where zombies eat people and only little pockets of bitter, dangerous humans survive. The zombies are reduced to being basic consumers. They walk, they kill, they eat. On the other hand, we see how intensely the survivors are living out their final days. They spend their time foraging and hunting for food. They live like our Cro-Magnon ancestors; their work is intrinsically connected to their survival. They are off the grid. They are outside the psychic crucible most of us live in each day. They are outside the chatter. They have no access to phones, computers, or TV, and if they did, they wouldn't mess with them anyway. They don't have the time. They live in the present.

The show is popular because it focuses on the important things, the essential things: food, water, shelter, and survival. The survivors want to live. The zombies only want to eat. Huxley's future humans are zombies, too. They shuffle through their lives in a narcoleptic daze, in thrall to a society that has destroyed the very concept of human dignity.

The question is: which side of the fence do you want to be on?

TRAPPED IN THE WEB

REFORM THE DEFORM

I pay special attention to pornography in this book. I'm young and formerly addicted. Older writers have, up to now, provided a lot of the interpretation of porn and the Internet. They write of pornography as a social and cultural construct. They are separated from the hard realities of never having known life without the Internet. To young adults, porn addiction is acute, painful, and deforming. Young adults have difficulty opening up to adults about pornography for fear of criticism, stigma, and shame. As a result, pornography is not given proper coverage in popular works about the Internet by authors like Sherry Turkle, Nicholas Carr, and William Powers, who have otherwise helped us better understand our relationships with the Internet.

Young people rely on the Internet and its unlimited supply of pornography to ward off external stress. The instant gratification gratifies instantly, soothing unquiet minds. But the external stress is, in large part, being caused by the Internet itself. The Internet is a feedback loop; it creates the demand that it then seeks to fill.

I'm all in. My personal reputation may be impacted by my public reckoning with the taboo topic of pornography, but it is important to me to help others who feel alone, confused, and helpless. I've been there. We have to talk about these things—porn use, sexual interaction with social media, and sexual dysfunction—openly and honestly, so that we can correct them to improve our lives.

I spent two years writing this. My first draft was over 400,000 words. I sacrificed. I toiled. I read. I wrote

A.T.

and wrote. People told me to wrap it up and then put it away in a coffin to rest. My friends thought I was crazy. It was an insane quest. I wrote this around the demands of classes and internship work and my first full-time job. I separated myself from people. I became a temporary recluse. It was clear early on that this book might hurt my career opportunities—at the very least in advertising technology, which is unfortunately the largest tech industry. My friends reminded me of the risks at every turn. But I felt motivated to press on. As Mary Anne Layden, psychotherapist and director of the Sexual Trauma and Psychopathology Program at the University of Pennsylvania, has asserted, "Once you know the truth, silence is complicity." After experiencing the pain of my dependencies and then reconfiguring my digital relationships and finding my life transformed, particularly from eliminating use of pornography, I knew I would never be silent again.

This book is a blueprint for understanding and reshaping your relationship with the Internet. I don't want to improve your life—I'm looking to save it.

TRAPPED IN THE WEB

PART I: THE INTERNET AND SOCIAL MEDIA

Separated from his product, man himself produces all the details of his world with ever increasing power, and thus finds himself ever more separated from his world. The more his life is now his product, the more he is separated from his life.

— Guy Debord

A.T.

Listen:

You are not a customer of Facebook, Snapchat, or any of the other social media websites. You are their chief product. This fundamental idea is key to understanding why social media websites work the way they do. If you learn nothing else from this book, remember this.

TRAPPED IN THE WEB

A BUSINESS NOT LIKE ANY OTHER

Social media services are for-profit companies that have responsibilities to their shareholders to maximize profits. The business of social media is advertising—developing advertising technology and capturing data from their users to make that technology even more effective, the advertising even more targeted. The more users social media companies have and the more time and attention those users pour into their services, the more user data they have to sell increasingly targeted advertising at a premium. For example, an entrepreneur from Kansas can market his new product to people from around the world with a particular subset of interests and traits (determined by their Facebook user data) that indicate they might be interested in his product. Social media allows advertisers to target particular demographics more quickly, precisely, and effectively.

In a fundamental way, the advertising technology created by social media companies enables a more efficient and precise exchange of information between businesses and consumers in a way that otherwise—in any other digital or non-digital realm—would not be possible on the scale that their advertising technology allows. This is economically meaningful and not necessarily a bad thing. However, it comes with a significant cost, not to Facebook and other social media companies, but to users like us, whom these companies rely upon to devote ever more attention and time to their services, allowing them to compile more and more data to sell more and more targeted advertisements.

It's a vicious circle.

A.T.

The grandiose claims that social media companies make about "connecting the world" are merely attempts to disguise their true goal of connecting more users to more businesses, to more advertisers burrowing even deeper into people's lives. The business model of social media is converting your bleary-eyed lost hours staring at screens into cash by exposing you to targeted advertisements. Siphoning off as much of your time as possible is the main agenda.

Social media employee stock options and ability to attain revenue growth goals depend on their continued ability to pump out cash, which all comes down to maximizing usage. There is a clear conflict of interest here. As users, we suffer from our obsessive and excessive use of social media—the very thing social media companies rely on. What's more, social media companies have the resources and technology to psychologically optimize their services to make them as addicting as possible. They are feeding off the addictions they create—a lucrative and destructive business model. Author Andrew Sullivan, in an aptly titled piece for New York magazine—"I Used to Be a Human Being"—described just what we are up against: "No information technology ever had this depth of knowledge of its consumers—or greater capacity to tweak their synapses to keep them engaged."[1]

Social media, like any other giant industry, has no conscience. The structure of the business is quite simple: keep users on their websites as long as possible, learn everything you possibly can about them, and then sell that information to other companies. The goal of social media websites is to keep you clicking; any human connection you might find along the way is incidental.

The psychological optimization that keeps you scrolling and clicking through websites is no accident. One tool that helps social media companies refine their websites is A/B testing, where companies test a design change by comparing the level of engagement with their service in a group exposed to the design change versus another group that wasn't exposed to the change. If the usage increases with the change, they roll out the new features. If not, they scrap them. Over time, this testing will become more and more automated; some services will morph on their own as they gain more data on user behavior and experiment with new features, colors, and placement of content.

Recently some teams have tried programming websites to visually morph based on inferences from user information so that they align better with the "cognitive style" of the user.[2] Based on your clicks and the information you accessed on the website, inferences made about you will automatically adjust the website. For services like Google Drive, design tweaks that personalize information and aesthetics based on user data could benefit users by reducing loss of cognitive resources when interacting with the interface. But for services like social networks and porn, where our emotional attachment is already high and it is already difficult to curtail excessive use, websites with adaptive designs may create an even more intense emotional engagement with users that may even further reduce our self-awareness and ability to normalize our use.

Here's one outcome of data-directed, psychologically optimized design: the new centralized feed of activity below the log out button on Facebook. To log

A.T.

out, you have to scroll to a very small icon in the top right-hand corner of the screen that is nestled just above a feed that shows you a list of all of your friends' current activity on Facebook—an additional barrier between you and your log out, your separation from Facebook—increasing the likelihood that you'll succumb to the temptation to donate more of your minutes and hours and days and weeks to the Facebook profit machine.

Enormous computing machines, mountains of money and data, and cutting edge, automated design is being wielded against us in the great battle for our time and attention. No wonder we're losing.

TRAPPED IN THE WEB

WE JUSTIFY WHAT IS SUCCESSFUL

Today in the U.S. we tend to build first, then monetize, and then try to philosophically justify what we create by marketing our creations. Snapchat is doing this right now with its public blog, which is populated by content from a PhD who has concocted compelling intellectual arguments that justify the "virtues" of our interaction with Snapchat. These blog entries are just sales copy dressed up in sophisticated rhetorical finery. Snapchat is not going to address or explore any potential consequences that might stem from the use of their product, nor are they going to be frank with their customers about their real agenda.

The build, monetize, justify model can be flawed because there are often deep, underlying costs that come with new technological developments that users and customers are simply unable to see in the moment. And companies trying to make money have no incentive to acknowledge or address these issues. In many cases, as discussed above, they have every incentive to amplify and profit from them. There's no referee. There's only more and more money as more and more of our lives are poured into the Internet.

A.T.

BEHIND THE EMERALD CURTAIN

I first began to understand all this during my work as a product manager intern at Nanigans, Facebook's venture-backed marketing partner. We created software that helped the largest companies spend billions of dollars in online advertising on Facebook with innovative tools and campaign optimization and performance tracking. The product managers are tasked with navigating the waters of the fast-changing, hyper-competitive adtech world and determining where to steer the development and design of Nanigans' software so that clients can more effortlessly and effectively spend more money through our platform.

This job led to conversations with Facebook's product team, which opened my eyes to the sophistication behind their data science and their ability to leverage data to make advertising more and more targeted, trackable, and effortless for advertisers. I was amazed by their advertising technology. I saw behind the emerald curtain. The wizard isn't a man. It's a vast panoply of awe-inspiring engineering.

Because all of our data is anonymized (we are nothing but user IDs in their advertising system) the algorithms and advertisers don't know any of our names, so I didn't feel concerned about privacy. But I was concerned about the conflict of interest between the social media companies and their users. The advertising optimization that produces the revenue that these social media companies are dependent on relies on users spending irrational, unhealthy amounts of time on social media, both to sell advertisements and to collect the data that optimizes them.

There's Scylla again. Scylla eats and eats and eats. It exists to eat. These social media sites exist to gobble up your time. This is their essence; this is what they do. Sometimes you can dance with Scylla and not get eaten. Sometimes you can use social media websites for something productive. But the danger to slip into the Internet vortex is always there. The Internet is pure appetite.

We are losing the battle; giant technocratic corporations are winning. In the face of the endless, boundless temptations that are instantly available to us, we often simply cannot exert the willpower and the energy necessary to resist. On Facebook, you are not a customer. You—your time, your attention, your friends, your clicks, your searches, your interests, your likes—are Facebook's product, a commodity to be bought and sold.

A.T.

WE ARE OUR USER DATA

Companies pay loads of money to have access to our data. Our data is our digital fingerprint, unique to us, revelatory. Companies mine our blogs, our video chats, our email. They sneak custom ads into our news feeds. They predict the videos we want to watch, the news stories that angle in our political direction. They have algorithms that predict the movies we want to watch, the music we want to listen to, the underwear that will make us look the best.

The online paradigm is predicated on human attention. Every website worth its salt is designed to keep you on that website just a bit longer. At its essence, the primary function of the Internet is to suck up your time, and, in so doing, create customer profiles for companies to sell to.

Our attention spans haven't evolved to handle the allure, the seduction, or the overload. Horror movies, by way of a strange example, scare us because movies have only been around a hundred or so years; what we see on the screen tricks us into thinking that we are the ones in danger even though we're safe at home on the couch.

The Internet does a similar thing. We feel connected to other people even though we aren't; we're safe at home, alone on the couch. News stories pop up and make us indignant; videos appear that make us laugh and cry. Book recommendations with the cheapest place to buy them pepper the edges of webpages. Movie previews of movies we want to see and didn't know existed pop up inside our web browsers. This might sound like a good thing, but it comes at a heavy price.

TRAPPED IN THE WEB

We trade our personal selves, our internal lives, to social media websites, which convert them into pure profit. In exchange, we are given the privilege of being sold things.

And with increased Internet speed and advancements in virtual reality technology, this is going to get a lot worse.

The current boom in entertainment technology—which will only continue to grow with the development of new technological platforms that provide more, and still more, stimulating entertainment—has grown in response to both the steep psychological costs of late-stage capitalism that it temporarily alleviates, as well as the abundance of free time that many people of privilege now have at their disposal. Robotics, automation, outsourcing—we are always looking for more free time, only to fill it with digital stimulation.

But here's the rub. Stimulation only leads to an appetite for further stimulation. Stimulation cannot satiate desire. The scratch just makes a bigger itch.

A friend of mine, a Brazilian student at Penn, transferred into a four-year dual degree program in engineering and business at Penn, which is one of the most challenging undergraduate programs in the world. He works out every morning. He meditates for 30 minutes every day. Both exercise and meditation have been shown to increase gray matter in the brain, which improves our ability to resist distractions. My friend has close to a 4.0 in the program, despite being a member of a social fraternity. He isn't a hermit. He is driven, ambitious, fit, and happy. How? We'll see.

A.T.

THE BRAIN IS A MUSCLE

Every generation gets the neuroses they deserve. Four hundred years ago, to give just one example, a relatively common mental illness was defined by the feeling that your limbs had turned to glass. Glass was rare and new, imbued with magical properties; a new technology became a concrete metaphor for how people saw themselves in the world. In the twenty-first century we are grappling with heightened rates of ADHD, depression, and suicide. ADHD and depression have a genetic component, but our environment, circumstances, and surroundings can also play an important role. The biggest recent change in our environment is our unhealthy dependence on digital technology, particularly repeated, acute artificial overstimulation from porn and repeated peer comparison via Facebook, Instagram, and the like. We can't change our genes, but we can change our technological environment.

We were the first generation to grow up with digital media. There may be a causal relationship between tech consumption and mental health. Author and neuroscientist Daniel Levitin provides a succinct set of statistics that shed light on our current state: "The suicide rate among middle-aged Americans increased by nearly 30 percent…according to a report from the Centers for Disease Control and Prevention. More than 10 percent of American schoolchildren, and nearly 20 percent of high-school-age boys, have been given a diagnosis of attention deficit hyperactivity disorder, and two-thirds of that group take drugs like Ritalin and Adderall to treat the condition."[3]

TRAPPED IN THE WEB

Young adults and children are most at risk for suffering the negative consequences of technology. Daniel Levitin explains: "Children are more likely to want immediate gratification, and they are less likely to be able to foresee the future consequences of present inaction; both of these are tied to their underdeveloped prefrontal cortices, which don't fully mature until after the age of twenty (!). This also makes them more vulnerable to addiction."[4] Children have shorter attention spans, a limited ability to exercise self-control, and fewer internal resources to cope with distraction, stress, disappointment, and the lure of instant gratification. Exposure to constant distraction and stimulation from digital media disrupts their intellectual development and their education.

Addiction to technology takes many forms, but porn is the most damaging. Without those fully developed prefrontal cortexes, young people, again, are particularly vulnerable to the negative consequences of pornography consumption: "Unlike adults, adolescents are believed to lack sufficient maturation and integrity in frontal cortices necessary to exert cognitive control required to suppress sexual cravings, thoughts, and behaviors elicited by pornographic content."[5] Their vulnerability extends beyond pornography: "There is also a small, but growing, body of research that indicates adolescents are increasingly struggling with compulsive Internet use (CIU) and compulsive behaviors related to Internet pornography and cybersex."[6] Young people's still-developing minds are malleable and easily influenced by the damaging content they don't yet have the self-control to resist. Other research agrees: "Teenagers;

brains are especially plastic. Now, 24/7 access to Internet porn is laying the foundation of their sexual tastes."[7]

Unlimited access to pornography is the hungry snake swallowing its own tail—desire begetting desire, a perpetual motion machine.

Like Huxley's future humans or the zombies on *The Walking Dead*, we are mostly oblivious to the consequences of our boundless appetites. The vast majority of us (including me, for far too long) incessantly engage with the Internet in ways that we have difficulty shaping and controlling. Some of the most competent people I have ever met are either completely oblivious to the damage they sustain from their unhealthy relationships to digital media or they are so attached to their behavior—the compulsive checking, scrolling, posting, and clicking—that they are incapable of correcting their unhealthy relationships. These people, who are fortunate enough to be competent despite adverse digital relationships, could be even more successful if they could recognize and confront their addictions to social media, pornography, and all manner of entertainment forever at their fingertips. Almost everyone is negatively impacted by their digital relationships, and even the smartest among us have difficulty identifying that and then doing the hard work to successfully correct those relationships.

TRAPPED IN THE WEB

THE PERMEABLE MEMBRANE

Popular culture never explores itself. It has no edges, no boundaries, no conscious will. What contours it might have are a permeable membrane. Pop culture has little shame, plenty of dark corners, and no real accountability. It is the collective amalgamation of all our tastes, our lusts, our preferences, our favorite movies and books and blogs and bands, and it is all manipulated by companies so large we can't really fathom them.

Porn is part of popular culture. Social media is a part of popular culture. The Internet is a huge engine of popular culture. YouTube sensations appear out of nowhere and end up with their own TV shows. The Internet has become the major staging ground for cultural products. But due to the nature of the Internet and the corporations that now dominate it, cultural products are not things you seek out and discover. Instead, they discover you; they seek you out.

The Internet advertises itself as a synonym for freedom. No one wants to question our digital dependencies because, almost overnight, we have marbled the Internet into every aspect of our lives—our bedrooms, our schools, our governing bodies. Unfettered access to the Internet has become sacrosanct.

Coverage of Internet dependency and addiction is scant given the pervasiveness of these issues. New technologies evolve at an increasing rate as more and more technologies are produced through endless re-combinations of old technologies, while our capacity to understand the implications of all of these new technologies does not evolve at pace. It's difficult to study or understand something while it is happening, and digital media is always in the process of happening.

Try to find an issue of *Time* or *American Century* from the 1950s. The articles are long, in-depth, complex, written in a direct but sophisticated style. You had to know things to understand them. A long attention span wasn't just expected, it was required. And these were popular magazines. Over the course of a few short decades, our attention spans have been drastically altered. Compare one of those old essays with an article in Time today. Now, everything is fast, short, simplified, and easy. We are dumbing ourselves down, and the Internet is more than happy to lend a helping hand.

In 2006, Mike Judge put out an interesting movie called *Idiocracy*. A regular guy from the early 2000s uses a time machine and wakes up in the far future. He discovers that he is now the smartest man alive. Humans have become supremely and decadently stupid. Everyone speaks in a slang so emptied of meaning that no one really says anything at all. The machines run themselves to the point that no one knows, or cares, how to operate anything. It isn't a great movie, but it is a damning satire.

We are marching into this weary vision of the future.

TRAPPED IN THE WEB

IT ISN'T ALL BAD NEWS

I should take a brief moment to focus on some of the benefits of social media. Some people, especially marginalized people, need access to human connection and interaction that isn't readily available in the flesh-and-blood world, and in some cases, the Internet can help. It's no substitute for real community, but it isn't nothing. Especially for people in very specific sub-groups—sufferers of certain rare diseases, aficionados of esoteric culture—or people who are isolated by geography, the Internet can offer real connection across time and space, the opportunity to know you are not alone in the universe even if you are alone in your room, your house, your school, your town, even your country. Especially for young people, this sense of connection can be essential to survival.

Social media can help expedite a transition from an "I" to a "We" culture. Facing existential threats like climate change and geopolitical instability, it's in our own self-interest to be more socially minded, working with others to find a way for humanity to continue to exist and thrive on this planet. Social media, in tandem with these global challenges that bring us outside the narrow scope of own limited individual desires, can help us develop a more community-oriented perspective and show us how we fit into a larger, inextricably interconnected world.

In a society where people move away from their families and communities all the time—for school, for work, for adventure, for fame or fortune—many of us are increasingly isolated from our loved ones. Social media can help maintain important connections between far-flung friends and family members, especially in times of crisis or disaster when people are frantic for news of loved ones.

Another undervalued benefit of social media is an extension of one of its creepier aspects. Social media companies optimize their services to gain ever more data to power their advertising systems, but this same data is helping us better identify and track criminals and terrorists—through the same data science technologies developed to improve the relevance of ads. This might be safety at a steep price, but for some, there is no price too dear.

Highlighting these benefits isn't a signal of my approval, but there is no avoiding the reality that we live in a world forever altered by social media. We need to figure out how to use social media for our benefit and jettison the rest.

TRAPPED IN THE WEB

THE MEDIUM IS THE MESSAGE

In the 1960s, philosopher Marshall McLuhan wrote about the consequences of electronic media overstimulation decades before the Internet was even a twinkle in the average American's eye. He memorably wrote: "I am in the position of Louis Pasteur telling doctors that their greatest enemy was quite invisible, and quite unrecognized by them." McLuhan's essential point was this: each new medium creates a different effect in the human mind. This effect is as important, if not more important, than the actual content the medium conveys. Content comes and goes, but the alteration of human minds through new media can change a society (almost) overnight.

Since the mid-century advent of television, no new medium has come close to the mind-altering potential of the Internet. It has altered the physical and psychic landscape of almost every country in the world. The Internet's effects on us—how it is shifting our attitudes and habits, the very fabric of our reality—are just now being noticed, studied, seen. The medium is the message, McLuhan cautioned.

To run with McLuhan's notion, I'll try to say it plain: when you are clicking around on the Internet, researching or playing video games or masturbating while watching porn videos, what you are actually doing is less important than what your interaction with the Internet is doing to you. Keep this in mind: using the Internet changes you.

No less a digital luminary than Steve Jobs saw the dangers. He prohibited his own children from using the very devices he was instrumental in creating. He knew that the Internet was addictive, that handheld devices were profound time-wasters. MIT professor Sherry Turkle explains how Silicon Valley employees, like Jobs, consciously seek to shield their children from the consequences of their creations: "Even Silicon Valley parents who work for social media companies tell me that they send their children to technology-free schools in the hope that this will give their children greater emotional and intellectual range."[8]

Those of us whose parents didn't have an inside track on the dangers of the Internet will have difficulty correcting our addictive relationship with the Internet because of habits that have been inculcated through years and years of repeated behavior. Long before I embarked on this book, I realized that my Internet overuse was adversely affecting me—I felt my personality disintegrating—but I struggled to make any changes because it had become such an ingrained part of my daily experience. I was habituated to the short-term benefits the Internet offered—the cheap thrills of likes and messages and comments and jerking off to porn—and ignored the longer-term costs—decreased productivity, decreased attention span, and mental health issues like depression and the fundamental loneliness that is both the fuel that feeds the social media machine and its ultimate product.

Correcting bad habits, especially Internet habits, is hard. The consequences we suffer are gradual and sometimes difficult to identify and attribute to our Internet use. This is particularly true for young adults whose whole lives have been shaped by the Internet.

Another obstacle preventing us from addressing our unhealthy dependency on the Internet is our herd mentality. We withhold judgment from certain behaviors because we (falsely) trust in the judgment of a large crowd. Even though our relationships to digital media cause us a lot of pain, it can be difficult to acknowledge this because our unhealthy relationships are shared by so many other people—seemingly *every* other person. But we have to look past the crowd to see ourselves. We have to challenge the new status quo.

A.T.

THE FEED

I was born in 1995. I grew up alongside the advent of new digital media during the early 2000s. I've never known a world without the Internet. I was connected to the World Wide Web before I went to school. I was in the first wave of students to see the impact that the Internet had on education. Rather than having access to information, data, and insight on how to best handle this new, suddenly ubiquitous technology, we were left to make sense of our digital relationships entirely on our own. Many of our parents and teachers, after all, understood the Internet less than we did.

Anyone born since, say, 1990 has been exposed to digital media during malleable, formative periods of their lives, so the consequences of their unhealthy digital dependencies are magnified. Not everyone my age sees it. Many of us love, or think we love, the amplified, plugged in, self-replicating digital reality. Others cannot envision a society different from the one we live in.

M.T. Anderson wrote about this in his dystopian novel, Feed. It's brilliant and terrifying. The novel begins in the near future, where everyone lives in the feednet, a vastly amplified Internet that people jack into directly in their minds. The feed, run by giant corporations, controls the information people can access. Virtual reality is so advanced that everyone prefers the feed to the real world—a radiated, near-ruin of dreary decay. The novel is disquieting in part because it reads like non-fiction, a report sent from twenty years in the future.

Imagine the Internet we actually use, only running twenty-four hours a day, inside your own retinas.

TRAPPED IN THE WEB

Implausible science fiction? Think again. Designers for multiple tech companies, including Google, are hard at work on this very concept. Google Glass was the first step. Think the feed is so far away? It isn't. It's a likely outcome of current trends.

A.T.

THE CENTRAL RECOMMENDATION

If you want a life outside the digital sub-reality; if you want to be productive, creative, and alert; if you want real relationships; if you want to be alive in the world, my central recommendation is this: disengage from the feed.

Disengage from pornography—today, right now—and other artificial sexual stimulation; disengage from fast-paced music constantly blaring through your headphones; disengage from fast-paced, jump-cut TV shows and movies with rapid scene-switching; disengage from video games, from dating apps, from unnecessary texting, and from news feed and profile browsing on social media. Cutting down on these behaviors is imperative.

Of course, disengaging from the Internet is easier said than done. Various feedback loops reinforce and perpetuate our relationship to computers. This is particularly true for introspective, introverted people like myself, whose perception of loneliness—which drives us to the Internet and is also fueled by the Internet—tends to be higher. The Internet is also the path of least resistance for those who are particularly vulnerable to the appeal of sexual stimulation afforded by interaction with social media and pornography. It can be hard to compete against our desires, which crave everything we know digital media can instantly afford. The challenge facing young adults today is that we have been dropped into a world of digital disinformation and sensory overload that tells us on a daily basis that pursuing our desires at all costs is the ultimate good. Only, it isn't.

My relationship with the Internet was not alleviating feelings of loneliness; it was amplifying my loneliness, bringing me to a state of frustrated depression. I felt boxed in, unable to breathe, trapped in an inescapable thought bubble of my own fucked up, addictive desires. I conditioned myself to need constant stimulation. I couldn't read, talk, study, or play the piano—all things that I love—because it all seemed too slow, too one-note. I couldn't drive my car without calling friends, texting at red lights, or toggling constantly between songs. I was always tired, yet always racing in a mad frenzy. I couldn't focus. I was anxious. I was vulnerable to a thousand distractions. I was unable to engage in solitude. My thoughts were a jumble. If I tried to check my yearning for my phone or laptop, my resistance would not last long, and I would feel more drained after my meager efforts. I was young and confused, yes, but also hopelessly addicted. I was in a low-fi version of Anderson's feed.

A.T.

WHAT DRIVES US TO INTERNET ADDICTION?

You must understand one important truth before we can go on. Internet use may feel like a harmless way of alleviating stress, but it isn't. The Internet is a highly addictive collection of time-wasting mental opiates. Its panoply of instant gratification and amped-up, airbrushed array of entertainment desensitize us to the real world, which increases our desire for more digital stimulation to relieve the stress of living with all that perceived dullness. (This is particularly true of pornography.) You need to cut off the source of this self-perpetuating feedback loop of stimulation and desensitization.

The medium *is* the message.

Are there factors that fuel our addiction to the Internet? Yes.

Alone? Bored? Depressed? Bothered by nagging, anxious thoughts? The Internet provides instantaneous access to near-infinite entertainment. The movies and video games and apps and porn temporarily distract us from our feelings of loneliness, melancholy, anxiety, fear, and despair, but they do not actually diminish those feelings. The distractions feel good in the moment. They feel like life, somehow. I know people who see the amalgamation of all these distractions as essential to their personalities. This is a grotesque deformation of the human condition.

But are we to blame? I don't think so.

The internal stress of being alone may be higher than it was in the past. The bulwarks of society—the webbing that held people together, the socially reliable institutions like the church, the family home, and long-term employment—are crumbling. Services like Facebook, Twitter, Netflix, and Pornhub have swooped in to fill the vacuum.

One of the major distinctions of American society for much of the twentieth century—a robust and thriving middle class—is disintegrating right before our eyes. There is an increased disparity between the wealthiest Americans and everyone else. As we well know, more and more wealth is being concentrated in the hands of the few while the many grow poorer.

Humans need work. We need things to do. And these things need to be connected to some survival function—the feeding of our loved ones, the preservation of our communities—or we suffer from the disconnect between our work and our purpose for living.

But what is that purpose? (Don't worry, I'm not going to even try to answer that one.) Part of the human odyssey, the journey each of us must make, is figuring this out for ourselves. What's one surefire way to make sure we aren't troubled with big, important questions about our purpose and how our work does or doesn't serve that? Digital distraction, served up hot, 24 hours a day, 365 days a year, even on Christmas.

It's not just meaningful work that eludes us here in the twenty-first century. We don't feel safe or secure. The geopolitical situation is dire. As of this writing, President Trump delivered an address to the United Nations threatening to annihilate North Korea. The specter of full-scale nuclear war has returned. There's a shortage of heroes, of belief in the public sphere, of faith in institutions. There's a paucity of optimism and a deluge of cynicism.

With all this uncertainty, people need their families, their work, and their communities. Yet we are now often separated from this succor, from the things that sustain us. Sherry Turkle wonders: "What are we missing in our lives together that leads us to prefer living lives alone together?"[9] In many cases, we are missing proximity to our loved ones.

New college students—suddenly flush with unstructured, discretionary time and without external regulations from parents or schools—have particular difficulty resisting the temptation to turn to the Internet to ease their loneliness, especially as they struggle to maintain a feeling of connection among widening, relocating, fragmenting social groups. Many college students join fraternities and sororities for connection to others. Many consume alcohol and drugs to combat the stress of finding themselves on their own for the first time in their lives. It's a scary, disorienting process, and digital media can serve as a soothing balm during the often lonely transition to adulthood. Or rather, it can feel like a balm. But it isn't.

I felt alone in the struggles and fears of a new life away from home. I was eighteen; I didn't realize how much I had relied on my parents until I was on my own. I turned first to alcohol—landing myself in the hospital during one of the first few weeks of school—and then to digital media to alleviate my loneliness and anxiety. But I found that my productivity plummeted, and I wasn't happy. Digital media was so immediately accessible, disguised as harmless social entertainment, and everyone was jacked into the Internet every day, all the time; it was the social norm. But it wasn't medicine. It wasn't a cure. The Internet was really a parasite feeding on, and growing, the loneliness I was trying to cure. A 2012 study at Columbia University found that the number of meals a family shares, a proxy for family togetherness, decreased the likelihood that young adults would use drugs.[10] Because social media and porn share many addictive qualities to drugs, it's not surprising that young adults deprived of that family togetherness, whether by divorce, by geographic separation, by smart phones, by careers that demand 24/7 availability, by financial hardship or parents who must work constantly to put food on the table, are drowning their sorrows in obsessive relationships with porn and social media.

Ultimately, though, it is not only college students and young adults who suffer from addiction to porn and social media. We are all trapped by the human condition, living out days that are numbered. Social media is a never-aging, never-dulling, never-sleeping fixed environment that is unaffected by climate change or political upheaval or sickness or sorrow. On social media we can shield ourselves from the cognitive pain inflicted by our environment by projecting ourselves onto profiles in an immortal, digital world—an alternative, ceaseless, infallible ether whose inhabitants never age, never sleep, and never lie awake at night fearing nuclear or climate apocalypse.

Digital media is a cheap, portable, instantaneously accessible means of combatting both the universal psychological pain of being human and the particular psychological pain of being young (or not young) and alone in the world. Internet porn, Facebook, Instagram,

Snapchat—these are the new opiates of the masses. New digital media collapses space and time, allowing us to ward off insecurities by remaining in a state of constant communication.

To be on the Internet is to be always and never alone. You might feel less lonely while you are connected to virtual friends or virtual sex, but the prolonged isolation from engaging with devices instead of people only intensifies and entrenches loneliness and depression. Sherry Turkle describes what quickly becomes a vicious cycle: "If lonely, you can find continual connection. But this may leave you more isolated, without real people around you. So you may return to the Internet for another hit of what feels like connection."[11] Digital connectivity is a middle ground between aloneness and togetherness, and this middle ground results in a paradox: technology that purports to connect users is also a drug that propels isolation. We produce cortisol—stress hormones—when we're alone for sustained periods of time. This stress might encourage us to reach for our phones or laptops, but the dopamine—a neurotransmitter that helps control our perception of pleasure—released in our brains when we engage with the addictive feedback loops of digital media only prolongs our state of isolation and prevent us from going out and reducing our cortisol levels through exercise, meditation, or human interaction. We use digital media more, we become more isolated, we become more stressed.

Everything about the Internet is self-perpetuating. The best representations are circles, repeating patterns, and loops. I keep thinking of a hamster, running in a wheel. The hamster runs and runs and never gets anywhere, but he doesn't know it. And neither do we.

Research from Carnegie Mellon that tracked Internet users over time suggests that Internet use may actually be a cause and not just a consequence of loneliness and depression. One professor concluded: "We were surprised to find that what is a social technology has such anti-social consequences."[12] Marshall McLuhan predicted a nation of "apathy and anxiety," and it seems that we've arrived at his grim future. Daniel Levitin writes, "Ours may be a time of material comfort and technological wonder, but it's also a time of aimlessness and gloom. During the first decade of this century, the number of Americans taking prescription drugs to treat depression or anxiety rose by nearly a quarter. One in five adults now regularly takes such medications."[13] Forms of new digital media all afford seductive, instantaneous stimulation—an effortless, temporary escape. Andrew Sullivan puts it this way: "Our phones are merely new and powerful antidepressants of a non-pharmaceutical variety."[14] But these new antidepressants offer no lasting solace. Whatever fleeting relief they provide is more than offset by the steep price they extract—hours, days, months of our lives lost forever to glowing screens. Huxley's future-humans. The walking dead.

A.T.

LEAVE YOURSELF ALONE

The numbers are staggering. A thorough study in 2009 found that the average person uses digital media for eight and a half hours a day.[15] A 2014 study conducted by University of Virginia psychologist Timothy D. Wilson found that students preferred receiving mild electric shocks to sitting alone with their thoughts.[16] In a 2015 study conducted by Microsoft, 77 percent of people ages eighteen to twenty-four agreed with the statement: "When nothing is occupying my attention, the first thing I do is reach for my phone." The same study found that more than half of participants aged eighteen to twenty-four admitted to checking their phones every thirty minutes or less.[17] According to Apple, in 2016 an average iPhone user unlocked their phone eighty times each day; an average Android user was found to unlock their phone 110 times a day.[18] A study at Nottingham Trent University in England found that young adults checked their phones an average of eighty-five times a day, which was twice what they had estimated. This amounted to an average of five hours a day spent on their phones.[19]

In an interview with Conan O'Brien, comedian Louis CK brilliantly but darkly exposes our aversion to solitude:

> You need to build an ability to just be yourself and not be doing something. That's what the phones are taking away—the ability to just sit there. That's being a person...Just be sad. Just let the sadness (come), stand in the way of it, and let it hit you like a truck...Because when you let yourself feel sad, your body has anti-

bodies—happiness that comes rushing in to meet the sadness...The thing is, because we don't want that first bit of sad, we push it away with a little phone or a jack-off or the food. You never feel completely sad or completely happy, you just feel kinda satisfied with your product, and then you die.[20]

When we let the pain of loneliness or boredom hit us like a truck, we strengthen our inner self and our ability to handle pain. In the process of confronting pain instead of escaping to a cellphone or a laptop, we also identify the goals and values that are important to us, which gives us purpose and motivation to overcome pain and move forward.

Constant access to entertainment trains us to expect constant and unlimited excitement. But life wasn't meant to be a non-stop carnival thrill ride. Philosopher Bertrand Russell explained in his 1930 book, *The Conquest of Happiness*:

> What applies to drugs applies also, within limits, to every kind of excitement. A life too full of excitement is an exhausting life, in which continually stronger stimuli are needed to give the thrill that has come to be thought an essential part of pleasure. A person accustomed to too much excitement is like a person with a morbid craving for pepper, who comes at last to be unable even to taste a quantity of pepper which would cause anyone else to choke. There is an element of boredom which is inseparable from the avoidance of too much excitement, and too much excitement not only undermines the health, but dulls the palate for every kind of pleasure, substituting titillations for profound organic satisfactions, cleverness for wisdom, and jagged

surprises for beauty...a certain power of enduring boredom is therefore essential to a happy life, and is one of the things that ought to be taught to the young.[21]

Solitude can be hard. Being alone is difficult. But over time we are able to transcend the initial pain and uncover a greater richness of experience—art, books, nature, in-the-flesh people, dreams for the future.

Bertrand Russell warned of the withering wrought by a life of constant stimulation: "A generation that cannot endure boredom will be a generation of little men, of men unduly divorced from the slow processes of nature, of men in whom every vital impulse slowly withers, as though they were cut flowers in a vase."[22] Boredom died when the Internet was born. We have to fight tooth and nail to reclaim it because without the inner self that only solitude can allow us to create, it's impossible to find and to be with the people and things that should be most important to us—family, friends, hobbies and passions, altruism, romance. How can we notice that hilarious, brilliant, sexy girl in math class if we've deprived ourselves of the opportunity to construct an inner self who can appreciate and pursue the virtues of a flesh-and-blood romantic interest?

Yes, the pain of solitude and boredom drive us to swipe and click the minutes away, but there are plenty of other push factors that make our fingers itch. Sherry Turkle prods us to ask: "Are we hiding from a good idea that will demand difficult work? Are we hiding from a question that will take time to sort through?"[23] We have to resist the temptation to avoid the short-term mental strain of work or a difficult task. Instead, we have to lean into the strain in order to avoid productivity loss from task switching or, even worse, losing sight of that game-changing idea or that important question. If we really need a break, we should take some time to decompress without digital media—go for a walk, do a few yoga poses, make dinner, call a friend—rather than engage with a digital distraction.

When we feel the impulse to use our devices, we have to ask what our motives are. If we're not avoiding hard work, is there something we really need to accomplish online, or are we running away from anxiety or stress or loneliness? When we can identify that we are turning to our devices to soothe our troubled minds, we can choose instead to suffer the temporary emotional pain of confronting whatever it is we seek to bury in porn or social media. We can address the source, the essential problem, deal with it, and move on. We then can reap countless long-term rewards by developing inner selves, cultivating our inner strength and emotional resources. We can become adults.

A.T.

THE TIME WARP

For all of recorded history, people have sought solace and relief from the stress and hardship of existence, especially during times of massive technological advancement and resulting societal upheaval. In his 1967 book *The Medium is the Massage*, Marshall McLuhan attests to the difficulty of adapting to such change: "Innumerable confusions and a profound feeling of despair invariably emerge in periods of great technological and cultural transitions."[24] To cope with the vast sea of changes wrought by eighteenth century industrialization and urbanization, people turned to zoos, parks, and pets. Now—as the world is remade once again—people turn to the light of tiny screens. Everyone needs distractions, entertainment, opiates to combat the anxiety of life on earth. While no opiate should be abused, reading, exercising, socializing with friends, playing an instrument, finding a new hobby or rediscovering an old one, are all far more satisfying alternatives to porn or video games or Facebook because they offer benefits and rewards in addition to short-term stress relief, and they do not have the longer-term costs of digital media abuse.

McLuhan presciently warned of a future that was then still decades in the distance: "These technologies will invade our inner peace, occupying our every waking moment. We will need a place to hide."[25] Creating a place to hide can be as simple as shutting off a phone, but sometimes we need a more secluded hiding place— the woods, a meadow, a creek, a beach, or even a city park. While I've had my share of cheap digital thrills, if I have lived at all it is because I have experienced blissful solitude in nature. We are part of nature. We are a product of nature. Just try it—surround yourself with green, with fresh air, with sky—and see if you don't feel that you can finally breathe again.

Every new technology, from the wheel to the telephone to the Internet, has forced humans to adapt—their minds, their relationships, and their values. New technologies that enhance and streamline our ability to exchange information, like all digital media, create a particular cognitive strain as we are bombarded with information at a staggering, ever-increasing pace. The result? Crushing, debilitating, desensitizing information overload. M.T. Anderson's feed.

The constant stream of information and stimulation flowing from all of our various devices devours our cognitive resources at an alarming rate. Instead of existing in our daily lives—observing, interacting, remembering—our minds are consumed by apps, notifications, updates, likes, tweets, texts, and on and on into the infinite digital horizon. Instead of living the minutes of our lives, we donate them to the hungry gods of the Internet, and days, weeks, months, and then years fly by unnoticed. Author Nicholas Carr writes, "When we're online, we're often oblivious to everything else going on around us. The real world recedes as we process the flood of symbols and stimuli coming through our devices."[26]

For me, this was a source of existential dread. When I was stuck in the feedback loop, things were moving too fast; there was nothing for me to hold on to, and though the years passed, I gained nothing in wisdom, understanding, or real experience of the world. I was blind to who I really was, to my interests and goals and dreams for the future. I moved around aimlessly, going through the motions in a digital time warp, my mind constantly occupied by that river of artificial stimulation from my ever-present devices. I was becoming de-personalized, de-realized. I felt my self-concept fragmenting, dissolving.

When I finally broke the feedback loop, controlled my relationship with digital media instead of letting it control me, I felt like Dorothy stepping out of black-and-white Kansas into Technicolor Oz. I was inhabiting my own life in a way I hadn't since I was a child. Without constant artificial stimulation, I began to engage with the world in a new way, gradually uncovering my inner self through solitude and introspection. The time warp, the existential dread, the fear that another unproductive year would be gone in the blink of a virtual eye—they all receded, and I was able to build relationships and plan for the future. My perception of time changed. It seems to move much more slowly now. I have more time and mental resources to absorb new information and process existing information. Days feel longer; weeks feel longer; I notice more; I remember more. I hadn't woken up with a dream at the cusp of my waking mind since I was a kid. Now that my subconscious mind is my own again, I wake with the swirl of dreams from the night before still making their way back to sleep.

Life is good. Or it can be.

TRAPPED IN THE WEB

THE TEMPTATION OF THE MULTI

But it wasn't easy.

We are infatuated, enchanted, entranced by novel visual information. We love to press our noses against the window of a car, a train, or a plane; we love to travel to distant lands or to undiscovered corners of our own cities. At its best, novel visual information challenges us to see things differently, to look at life with fresh eyes. With digital media, there's no need to hop in a car or a plane or even to walk across town—novel visual information is now only a click and a scroll away. With endless content—TV shows, movies, video games, pornography—at the tips of our fingers, we can mainline novelty from the comfort of our own beds. Nicholas Carr writes, "The natural state of the human brain, like that of the brains of most of our relatives in the animal kingdom, is one of distractedness. Our predisposition is to shift our gaze, and hence our attention, from one object to another, to be aware of as much of what's going on around us as possible."[27]

Multitasking has become so ubiquitous that it almost seems silly to name it. What was once notable—working on multiple tasks at one time—is now standard operating procedure. Research has shown that what often motivates multitasking is the desire to perceive oneself as being productive. Unfortunately, and paradoxically, multitasking is wildly unproductive. A 2012 study from Ohio State University found that multitasking didn't actually help people be more productive.[28] The conscious mind can only do one thing at a time. By multitasking, you are actually dividing up your mental energies into tiny allotments, constantly refocusing the brain on a new task, never completing the first one. It's a silly way to do anything. Imagine cooking a meal. You cut a little piece of carrot, then run over and start chopping a potato. You julienne a few wedges of potato and then go and put a little salt on a filet of salmon. You slice a lemon, stopping in the middle, and return to the carrot. This is no way to make dinner. Or to live your life.

Earl Miller, a neuroscientist at MIT, explains that people were "not wired to multitask well... When people think they're multitasking, they're actually just switching from one task to another very rapidly. And every time they do, there's a cognitive cost in doing so."[29] Daniel Levitin explains the science behind this "cognitive cost": "Asking the brain to shift attention from one activity to another causes the prefrontal cortex and striatum to burn up oxygenated glucose, the same fuel they need to stay on task. And the kind of rapid, continual shifting we do with multitasking causes the brain to burn through fuel so quickly that we feel exhausted and disoriented after even a short time. We've literally depleted the nutrients in our brain."[30]

The feeling of productivity we have when we multitask is misleading, particularly when we are checking social media for notifications. It can feel like a productive distraction. It's not. This is not real productivity; this is vanity productivity. It is similar to pursuing "vanity metrics," when startup teams optimize for the less important, short-term, instantly attainable "wins", like finding and sending emails to investors and getting a certain number of likes on a Facebook page, instead of focusing on the more challenging, important metrics of sales and revenue growth.

Before cellphones and the Internet, there were higher barriers to communication, and there was more predictability to that communication—the mail came once a day; you had to be in the house to hear the phone ring. There was more undistracted time to engage in solitude and work without the pressure and anxiety of constantly wondering who was trying to get in touch, who might be waiting for a response. Now our phones are always at our fingertips, and we are always waiting, always watching, which erodes our ability to engage in focused work.

William Powers, author of *Hamlet's Blackberry*, writes: "By some estimates, recovering focus can take ten to twenty times the length of the interruption. So a one-minute interruption could require fifteen minutes of recovery time. And that's only if you go right back to the original task; jam other tasks in between and the recovery time lengthens further."[31] According to a study by Microsoft tracking email behavior of twenty-seven employees, it took workers an average of twenty to twenty-five minutes, on average, to return to their work at full focus after being interrupted by an email or instant message, attesting to the cognitive "tax" levied by distraction, which we are all vulnerable to because of our constantly connected lives.[32]

As if all of that wasn't enough, multitasking is a compounding force, increasingly eroding focus. Every time you task switch you drain cognitive energy, which reduces the cognitive energy available to resist future distractions, which increases the likelihood of task switching again in the near future, leading to more task switching and then more vulnerability in a vicious negative feedback loop. To make matters worse, the novelty of task switching provides a short-term dopamine kick. But this only drains more cognitive energy, reducing your ability to pay attention for a sustained period of time without seeking dopamine from task switching with other distractions. This can quickly degenerate into a state of continuous distraction, where you are never able to work for more than a minute or two at a time.

 The energy drain from our lifestyles of continuous multitasking is one reason why some of the most extreme cases I've encountered need excessive amounts of coffee and Red Bull to get through the day. One friend kicks things off by waking up and reaching his hand across to the bedside table, where a caffeine cube is waiting. This guy is one of the smartest people I know, with a 2400 on the SAT, but during lectures, I noticed that he was constantly shifting between checking email, texts, Facebook, Hacker News, Politico, his fraternity Slack group, a paper he was writing, and some coding assignments, all while attempting to listen and take notes. It was insane. He was burning the midnight oil, brain-wise, melting down the candle on both ends. If he had eliminated continuous multitasking and let the mental economies of scale kick in from focusing on a singular task for a sustained period of time, he would have been much more effective while using much less energy. He would have been happier, too.

 Young professionals often buy into the work hard, play hard lifestyle. But most people tend to work more and play less. We may think that we're striking some coveted work-life balance by having our phones with Facebook, Snapchat, Instagram, and text messages running a constant drumbeat of potential "play" throughout our working days, but this incessant juggling of work and social interaction results in substantial productivity loss, destroying almost all the time we have to actually play in the real world.

Even something as innocuous as checking your email impacts your day. Continuously checking email fragments attention and inhibits your ability to engage in productive, sustained, and, especially, creative work. When you're constantly checking your devices, your mind becomes "reactive," especially as you send out more texts or emails or Facebook comments. Then you're expecting the next message and wanting to respond immediately, but you never know when that next message will arrive, so you're allocating untold mental resources to constantly anticipating its arrival so you can respond right away. This reduces the amount of mental resources we have available to focus on what matters, which makes us less productive, even less intelligent.

Research out of Hewlett-Packard in 2005 by Glenn Wilson identified that the IQ scores of knowledge workers fell from their normal level by an average of ten points—twice the 4 point decline observed for those smoking marijuana—when distracted with emails or texts.[33]

A.T.

RESISTANCE ISN'T FUTILE

I recommend several behavioral changes in order to disengage from lifestyles of constant Internet multitasking.

Whenever possible, eliminate digital social interaction while working. This requires physically separating from devices. The problem is not just the amount of time we spend distracted on our devices. The problem is also the amount of energy we need to spend *fending off* the constant desire to distract ourselves on our devices, especially when they are on hand, which magnifies the temptations. But that being said, it's often hard to put our phones away before studying at the library; we are so reliant on the temporary stimulation of digital media that separation from our devices causes mental pain, actually making it initially *harder* to study than if we were multitasking on our devices. But over time it becomes more tolerable, and the productivity gains are well worth the initial discomfort.

One in three teenagers sends one hundred text messages a day, and 15 percent send more than two hundred a day, which adds up to six thousand texts a month.[34] Forty-one percent of teens with cell phones said that they would describe themselves as "addicted" to their phones, according to Common Sense Media.[35] As a student and as an intern at a Facebook partner, I realized that my texts, emails, and messages were rarely extremely time sensitive (and even those that were could usually wait for a few hours). Once I restricted my digital communications to a few discrete periods—I recommend three—throughout the day, I experienced an immense surge of productivity. To avoid any potential cost to relationships in a society where we've been conditioned to expect immediate responses, consider setting an automatic text and email response informing people that you will be responding to their messages later. Daniel Levitin suggests this: "I will try to get to your e-mail within the next week. If this is something that requires immediate action, please telephone me. If it still requires my reply and you haven't heard from me in a week, please resend your message with '2nd attempt' in the subject line."[36]

Avoid the temptation to check email and texts first thing in the morning. Every time I succumb to the urge to reach for my phone immediately after I wake up I end up spending the rest of the morning thinking subconsciously about how to respond to the messages I've received, which interferes with my productivity and focus at work. If there are no messages waiting for me first thing in the morning, I end up checking my texts and emails more frequently throughout the day to alleviate worry about why no one's contacting me.

When writing emails, especially for work, you should be concise and fast. Author William Powers suggests you keep your emails to no more than five sentences; this strategy will make email-writing quick, effective, and less daunting. There is no need to waste time and intellectual resources in making what should be informal communication more formal than it needs to be.

Multitasking can also take the form of listening to music, watching TV shows or movies, or playing video games while working. Daniel Levitin explains why this doesn't work: "Russ Poldrack, a neuroscientist at Stanford, found that learning information while multitasking causes new information to go to the wrong part of the brain. If students study and watch TV at the same time, for example, the information from their schoolwork goes into the striatum, a region specialized for storing new procedures and skills, not facts and ideas. Without the distraction of TV, the information goes into the hippocampus, where it is organized and categorized in a variety of ways, making it easier to retrieve."[37]

Everyone needs a mental vacation here and there—try daydreaming for a break instead of reaching for your phone. Daniel Levitin explains: "The natural intuitive see-saw between focusing and daydreaming helps to recalibrate and restore the brain. Multitasking does not." Go for a walk, meditate for five minutes, read a book—you might even find that ideas, solutions, and innovations emerge while you're productively disengaged from work. Books are medicine for the brain. The human mind is hardwired for narratives.

I get it. We all want, even need, to be distracted sometimes. Smart distractions can be utilized as a tool to ward off the temptation to turn to productivity-sucking distractions like email, Facebook, porn, etc. For instance, listening to repetitive, slow-paced music (ideally nature sounds or instrumentals) on low volume while working can help you resist temptations to do other things, allowing you to focus more completely on your work. One ADHD sufferer I interviewed attested to the value of engaging in a lesser distraction to resist greater distractions while working: "I would knit during lectures so that I could maintain focus in my head."

You can also try working at a standing desk. The same ADHD sufferer said: "In my boarding school different kids could use different kinds of stimulation—they would work while standing up so they could move around occasionally because when you're sitting down there is absolutely no ability to distract yourself from the conversations in your head. A little bit of physical stimulation, like wiggling the feet around or stretching or temporarily moving around, is good."

Lifestyles of continuous multitasking encourage a state of continuous partial attention—subconscious multitasking—where the mind, conditioned to expect constant interruption and task switching, never fully focuses on one task. Many people who engage heavily with social media, dating apps, and digital social communication—anything that conditions users to be constantly on the alert for responses—suffer from continuous partial attention. Describing this state of continuous partial attention, the *Harvard Business Review* explains: "We keep the top level item in focus and scan the periphery in case something more important emerges. Or something more alluring, reassuring, or simply less demanding."[39]

In order to succeed and accomplish difficult goals, rather than constantly multitasking and living in a state of continuous partial attention, you need to be able to focus on singular tasks for sustained periods of time. "People," Nietzsche says, "whose thinking is active in one direction" achieve great things.

You have to find meaning in your work. You have to find beauty in it. You have to find passion and enthusiasm; without it, you are lost. The best way to find meaning in your work is to sensitize yourself to stimulation by minimizing time spent with devices and increasing solitude and introspection. People who are sensitive to stimulation, who are able to be captivated by activities that aren't inherently or obviously stimulating, can have sustained focus on singular tasks for sustained periods of time without needing to expend energy resisting distraction. This is how the most innovative, complex, and creative ideas are incubated. This is how the best work is completed. Sensitivity to stimulation allows people to notice the seemingly insignificant, to tolerate boredom and solace and reflection, which are absolutely essential for having creative realizations, restoring energy, and identifying an inner voice. If we don't give our minds the space they need to do really good, really hard work, how can we succeed at anything we truly care about?

TRAPPED IN THE WEB

MUSIC CAN BE THE ENEMY

Music is good for your brain and your body. Listening to music can lower blood pressure and anxiety and improve mood and memory. Listening to the right music, as discussed above, can help you focus on your work and resist the temptation to fragment your attention with social media or another time-wasting distraction.[40] We just have to be sure that we're not using music as yet another multitasking crutch—a way to avoid the pain of hard work and concentrated effort or of solitude and silence. The headphones of today allow us to immerse ourselves in concussive, near-total sound. I know people who listen to music while walking, driving, fishing, skate-boarding. They listen to music while working, playing sports, having sex. I like music, but it can be just another thing to get lost in, especially when the interface is our phones, iPads, or laptops.

Acclimation to constant audio stimulation makes it difficult to engage in quiet tasks like reading, working, and reflecting. Every religion preaches that the divine communicates to us through silence. Don't be afraid of it.

Listening to music for stimulation while studying or working deprives you of the opportunity to summon interest in your work from within—often by connecting your work to longer-term goals in order to gain enough energy to combat the draining nature of the work. And if you are unable to generate sufficient interest to energize yourself to get work done without music, then you'll be forced to find other solutions, like actually taking that needed nap, doing squats or some push-ups, or drinking a cup of coffee.

I believe music is good for the soul. But constant music is too much of a good thing. It creates another feedback loop where the normal state of affairs, the equilibrium we're always seeking, is sound filling our ears.

Given our dependence on frequent overstimulation, it's no wonder that young adults listen to music while studying, going to class, eating, going to the bathroom, and working out; we have worn down our dopamine receptor sensitivity from repeated acute overstimulation from pornography, and this makes normal life feel dull and colorless. We seek to negate the dullness of life outside pornography by consuming another layer of artificial stimulation through music.

The solution is definitely not to avoid music altogether. But if you're using it to fill important and possibly productive silence, skip it. Instead of listening to music between classes, I recommend that students try to recall two to three things that were of interest or particular importance from the previous class. This will help develop a strong understanding of those two or three concepts. If you do this after every class instead of listening to music, by the time exams roll around you will have a much stronger understanding of many of the core concepts of your classes. Studying for exams can then be a genuine effort to reinforce and expand your understanding of the course material, rather than a frantic cram session. You will be a better student and a more interesting person.

Associating different kinds of music with different tasks can allow you to improve the efficiency of mentally switching between those tasks. For instance, if you come to associate a certain kind of music with partying, you can listen to that kind of music before going out to help transition your mind from work to socializing. Similarly, if you come to associate a certain kind of music with certain kinds of work, you can listen to that music to give your mind a cue to transition from socializing to work. This can also apply to switching between different kinds of work.

A.T.

AIM FOR THE FLOW

Flow is a state of high productivity that comes from focusing on a singular task for a sustained period of time without distraction. Psychologist Mihaly Csikszentmihalyi, who recognized and named the concept, believes "flow" comes from undisturbed focus on a single, challenging, but completable task (or completable portion of a task) and results in the immense cognitive reward of not only heightened productivity, but also greater happiness.

Having a device on or near you puts you in a reactive state that impedes the ability to fully immerse yourself in your work, as your mind will be subconsciously worrying about whether or not it will be distracted and pulled out of "flow," which prevents it from fully engaging in "flow." As the ancient playwright Seneca said, "To be everywhere is to be nowhere."

Symptoms of ADHD can be environmentally induced, driven by our relationship to our digital environment. Dimitri Christakis, professor of pediatrics at the University of Washington in Seattle, found that the increase in rates of ADHD over the last twenty years might be at least in part attributable to environmental factors like "the fragmented, action-packed nature of digital media."[41] One person with biological ADHD attested to the widespread nature of what she believed to be environmentally induced ADHD: "Everyone struggles with distraction issues. It's hard to be forced to be interested in everything, for extended periods of time."

Even Microsoft, in a 2015 report, recognized the

decline in attention span from our interaction with our digital environment. It was removed from the Internet, but beforehand, publications covered it: "A recent study from Microsoft Corporation has found this digital lifestyle has made it difficult for us to stay focused, with the human attention span shortening from 12 seconds to eight seconds in more than a decade."[42] A goldfish has an attention span of nine seconds. And if that doesn't rattle you to your very core, then you're already lost to the hamster wheel.

The brilliant friend who started each day with a caffeine cube was suffering from environmentally inflamed symptoms of ADHD. He had a deep addiction to multitasking, and his reduced productivity was incompatible with success or sanity at Penn. One late Sunday evening (technically it was very early Monday morning), he hit rock bottom. He began pacing outside our dorm, roaming around the giant structure. Something broke inside him. He kicked down the back door and stormed into the dorm, wailing, tears streaming down his face, yelling, "I can't do it all! I can't do it all!" Everyone in the dorm awoke and ran downstairs. We found him chugging a bottle of booze; he was trying to drink himself to death. We tried to calm him down while someone called the police. They took him to the nearby Penn hospital.

Though ADHD can be combatted with pharmaceuticals like Ritalin and Adderall, these drugs have negative side effects like anxiety and irritability; they're addictive, and they have incredible potential for abuse. Those with environmentally induced symptoms of ADHD should avoid prescription drugs and instead

A.T.

focus on reshaping their relationships with digital media. Even for those who require medication for managing symptoms of ADHD, restricting use of digital media and working hard to avoid multitasking will still be incredibly beneficial.[43]

TRAPPED IN THE WEB

THE ITCH THAT CAN'T BE SCRATCHED

A big driver of all this multitasking madness is social media. Remember, social media isn't there to make you happy and fulfilled; it exists to siphon off your happiness as a product for private companies. You are not a patron or customer of social media sites; you are their bread and butter.

Social media is all about feedback loops. One person I interviewed has one he calls "getting stuck." After spending too much time on his phone, he feels anxious and guilty, and then he spends more time on his phone, flooding himself with new information in order to drown out those feelings.

Digital media scratches the itch that it creates.

In some ways *all* of the internet is a series of these loops: social media, advertising, movie clips, message boards. They create artificial need, artificial hunger.

When we consume the news feed, the social anxiety from subconscious comparison makes us more vulnerable to ads: to clicking ads and buying products and services marketed *to reduce social anxiety*. This is why many see clothes advertised on Facebook (and Instagram, which Facebook owns). Like uploading content and receiving external validation, purchasing cool new clothes (or other things) increases our sense of status and reduces social anxiety created from peer comparison on the news feed.

The news feed creates a need for the news feed and the products in the ads. It's diabolical. People often don't realize they are being sold to when they are scrolling through their news feed. The ads often feel spontaneous, and as they are often matched up with our profiles, we already lean towards the products we're being sold.

We're vulnerable, and because of this vulnerability, advertisers spend more. Facebook can price ads higher, making more money per ad. Facebook can track this and price it, because Facebook is not only able to track clicks, but also purchases after clicks. And even if you don't purchase right after clicking an ad—if you make a purchase of that company's product a few weeks later, Facebook can still attribute that (through cookies). And they deserve to, from a business sense, because the ad subconsciously impacted you, particularly in your state of vulnerability, and probably helped inform that later decision in purchasing a product.

We use Facebook, feel insecure and inferior, and are influenced by ads and buy things marketed to reduce those negative feelings and give status. Or, we upload more glorified, romanticized content for external validation, which makes others feel insecure and inferior. Facebook makes money. We spend money, often to recoup our sense of self worth.

Facebook ads are damningly, maddeningly effective. They *work*. Using the data we've given them, they sell us products based on that data. And due to manifold forces I've already outlined, we are exposed prey.

In the late nineteenth century, William James wrote, "The deepest principle in human nature is the desire to be appreciated." Young people spend so many hours and so much money at bars and nightclubs because the desire to be social and to be desired as a social companion is an incredibly powerful, motivating, even obsessive force. The magnitude of this force explains the popularity of social media, which takes the fraternity, the bar, the coffee shop, and the party and puts them into a portable, nonstop desire machine. Who could possibly put that down?

There is a feedback loop of sexual anxiety that drives social media use—who wants us; how can we make them want us more; who do we want; who else might we want? There is no end to the wanting and the worrying when Facebook puts a whole world of our peers—curated to the nines—constantly at our finger-tips. As one person I interviewed told me: "If I had Facebook, if you were into a chick, you would look at her page and think, 'Wow, I need to look at her to remind myself that is what I'm going for, and this is how much better it would be if I was with her and not jerking it.'" But you're not with her; you're on Facebook. But you're turned on by her photos, and before you know it, you've clicked over to porn. Now you've masturbated, reducing energy and motivation, leading to more isolated consumption of pictures on Facebook, dreaming of a way out of the porn vortex with some of those real girls.

But those "real" girls—how real are they? Social media allows us to romanticize and glorify ourselves; we can all seem flawless and limitless—"Penn face," everyone called it when I was in school, the perfect façade. This feigned perfection not only requires constant, obsessive attention to maintaining and cultivating our profiles, not only eats away at the self-esteem of all of our "friends" who view the product of our prodigious labors and deem themselves less worthy, it also destroys the age-old allure of meeting a new romantic interest—mystery. Constant

A.T.

access to these idealized, ridiculous versions of each other destroys opportunities for us to develop the mysterious, enchanted attractions that allow people to fall in love. Instead of clinging to a romantic memory from a first encounter, embellishing it in our imagination to form an enchanted understanding of a new love interest, we have information to access. With boundless information comes the death of mystery. Without mystery, without room for imagination, there is no enchantment.

I know this from personal experience. Access to information on social media drained my motivation to date. Why try to get to know someone if everything you'd ever want to know about her is right there on her Facebook page? Why spend the time to discover that a girl has a killer laugh or that the way she pushes her hair out of her eyes makes your legs turn to jelly if you can view five to five hundred photos of her on Facebook and determine that she's not actually that hot? McLuhan anticipated that a social network based on image sharing would commoditize the self, reducing the subjective infatuation our imaginations and our hearts can concoct and develop for one another: "Both monocle and camera tend to turn people into things, and the photograph extends and multiplies the human image to the proportions of mass-produced merchandise."[44]

We create ourselves as objects on Facebook, and we consume others as objects on Facebook. We become mass-produced merchandise. We have commodified our desires, objectified our wants and needs. Nothing is private. Every dream or want or kink is now part of a new Internet currency, where sharing is expected and privacy is kitsch. Everything is for sale.

All those hours we spend scrolling through the carefully composed, completely objectified lives of our digital friends and perfect strangers exact their toll in insecurity and inferiority, comparison, envy, and self-doubt. What better way to alleviate all of that social anxiety than to upload new content to Facebook or Instagram and monitor that content for those precious "likes" and "hearts"? Who knows when that validation will arrive? We'd better monitor that content quite closely. While we're monitoring, we might notice that another "friend" has, in the meantime, uploaded some new, enviable content. And so goes the feedback loop of social anxiety.

This feedback loop cycles between two main axes: social anxiety from peer comparison and the reduction of social anxiety from external validation. Unfortunately, peer comparison and self-esteem that is closely tied to external validation contribute to symptoms of depression. This may be one reason why a recent long term study showed increased use of Facebook contributed to reduced mental health and life satisfaction.[45] While Facebook calls itself a social network, it might be more apt to think of it as a system, a factory for producing and reducing anxiety through the forces of peer comparison and external validation. If there is any satisfaction from using Facebook, it is the satisfaction of alleviating the social anxiety produced by using Facebook. Social media, including but not limited to Facebook, is like a video game involving the loss and recuperation of confidence. But every time that confidence is lost and then recuperated on social media we erode our internal, stable self-esteem and emerge with a sense of self-worth

A.T.

that is increasingly superficial and dependent on the clicks of virtual strangers.

TRAPPED IN THE WEB

THE PROGRAM: REDUCING YOUR RELIANCE ON SOCIAL MEDIA

I have ascetic tendencies. My digital diet was extreme. I don't advocate such tough measures for everyone, but I do think considering a digital diet for yourself is useful and wise. My digital diet involved using social media less (by eliminating social media notifications, uploading less content, and having fewer "friends" on social media), listening to slower-paced instrumental music, and ignoring click bait and political articles, which tend to simply produce empty dopamine and arousal. I staggered and limited the time I spend checking email, texts, messages on Messenger, and phone calls. I also eliminated TV and movies entirely, unless I'm with friends or family. I know it's extreme, but I like who I am when I'm not spending my free time consuming hours and hours of novel visual entertainment.

I followed one diet. There are others. The program I outline here aims to reduce social media use, which was the most important component of my digital diet—the change that I would urge you to adopt first. A reminder: I'm not advocating that we eliminate social media altogether. That way lies paranoia, anxiety, and existential isolation. I'm not a Luddite. The Internet isn't evil, just misused.

A quick outline of the program:

1. Eliminate use of notifications.
2. Have a few great photos.
3. Have a minimal friend list.
4. Eliminate news feeds and scale back on profile browsing.

A.T.

5. Separate yourself from your phone as often as possible.

TRAPPED IN THE WEB

STEP ONE: ELIMINATE USE OF NOTIFICATIONS

Ivan Pavlov famously discovered that dogs began to salivate when they saw objects they associated with food. They evolved to salivate when they ate, but they learned to salivate when the lab assistant, who always brought them their food, appeared. Pavlov began to experiment with different associations and confirmed that responses that were considered innate could be conditioned. Dogs could be trained.

People can be trained, too.

Pavlov's experiments help shed light on our obsessive relationship with Facebook notifications. He demonstrated that randomized rewards, rather than continuous or regular rewards, are the best way to reinforce reward-seeking behavior. If we never know when we'll be rewarded, we're better off seeking that reward all the time, just in case. We are obsessed with Facebook notifications, in no small part because they arrive at randomized, unpredictable intervals.

Remember: the medium *is* the message.

I wouldn't be surprised if Facebook and other social media companies figured out ways to give more and more notifications, algorithmically programmed to be unpredictable, to be as variable and cognitively obsessive as possible. I was imprisoned by this ingenious system of variable reward, losing time, focus, energy, and sleep, working much less inefficiently. Then, lightning struck. What if I ignored my notifications? Would the sky fall? When I didn't check my notifications on Facebook, they would gradually climb to ninety-nine and then revert back to zero. Rather than continuously

A.T.

oscillating between work and social media, monitoring my notifications, I was able to use Facebook more purposefully and selectively. Over a year-long span of not checking notifications, I did not miss out on any important information. Yes, I probably missed a few comments and updates of who liked my pictures, but those are digital interactions that I was well rid of. I almost missed an event that was exclusively planned through Facebook without any other verbal, physical, or email invitation, but, as luck would have it, two hours before the event, my friend mentioned the party, his girlfriend's, at the gym, and I was able to attend. The universe smiles upon those who ignore notifications. Trust me. You do not need this feature in your life.

Disengage from notifications. They do nothing, and they take a lot in exchange.

TRAPPED IN THE WEB

STEP TWO: HAVE A FEW GREAT PHOTOS

I used to spend my time at parties wondering: When can I take a photo that, if uploaded to social media, would allow me to capture social value on my profile? I worried that someone else would post a picture first, or post a better picture, and get all the social cache from that party, and then all the time I'd spent at the party, which was entirely devoted to worrying about that photo, would have been wasted. It's an old problem—spending more time trying to record an experience as opposed to *just experiencing* it—with new dimensions. Once upon a time, our parents or our grandparents might have made a choice about photographing or videotaping a special event—a birthday party, a recital, a holiday, or a family vacation—or giving it their full, in-the-moment attention. But now, thanks to digital cameras and camera phones and Instagram and Facebook, every mundane moment is something we might capture for Internet posterity.

Those of us who have grown up using social media are constantly seeking to convert moments in the real world into social capital. The new defining mantra: "I am seen therefore I am." Constantly directing mental resources to thinking about what content to share and constantly uploading that content and monitoring it for validation is stopping us from engaging in the real world. And it's also not the best way to create the most attractive profile.

Having a few *great* photos, rather than constantly uploading endless mediocre photos to a vast library of images, may actually make you look more attractive and more desirable. The quality of those few photos will be higher. There's more room for someone's imagination to take hold and be enchanted by you. And, most importantly, having only a few photos makes you look like someone who is happily engaged with the living of a real-world life and not in need of constant external validation. You'll also save a ton of time and mental resources not worrying about the need to upload more photos, so this step is a win all around.

Look: I'm not a monk or a prude or a hermit. I still maintain accounts, and occasionally I upload content to market myself socially and sexually. But it isn't an obsessive time-waster. I am in complete control.

I knew a guy once, by way of example, who only owned ten shirts. When he bought a new one or received one as a gift, he would give one away. He did this to simplify his life and his wardrobe choices. He always looked fashionable because he didn't hold on to old clothes. So: don't have more than ten photos—simplify and always look fashionable.

TRAPPED IN THE WEB

STEP THREE: HAVE A MINIMAL FRIEND LIST

Just as it is difficult to focus on reading or writing when you're in a public, social space like a dining hall or bar, it is difficult to focus on reading or writing when you maintain an expansive digital profile in the massive, public, social space that is social media. The more friends you have to distract you on Facebook the more time you'll spend distracted on Facebook. It's that simple. It's a question of energy. Facebook likely knows this, and it is why the website is constantly recommending new friends.

I have under 300 "friends" on Facebook. One way to determine who to keep as a friend and who to remove is to consider whether or not you would initiate a conversation with a digital "friend" you ran into on the street; if you wouldn't at least say "hello," then remove that friend. I brought my friend count down despite being in a fraternity, having been on a varsity sports team, and having worked in various technology companies, and while I accept new friend requests and add more "friends" based on new, real relationships, I periodically review my friend list and delete friends that are no longer a part of my life.

Don't think about it in terms of other people's feelings. If you care about them at all, you should communicate with them from time to time. If you aren't communicating with them, do yourselves both a favor and remove them from your friend list.

A.T.

**STEP FOUR: ELIMINATE NEWS FEEDS AND
SCALE BACK ON PROFILE BROWSING**

Do this today without a second thought: delete social media apps on your phone. You can begin to restore control over your life and your relationships with this simple step.

Delete the apps for Instagram, Snapchat, and Facebook—all of the social networking apps on your phone. Keep the Facebook Messenger app, which gives you the benefit of instantaneous communication without sucking you into the black hole of news feed and profile-browsing that does nothing for you other than make you anxious, envious, irritated, or all three at the same time.

If you must keep the social media apps on your phone, and I really think you should get rid of them, I recommend eliminating push notifications from those apps. Unlike Messenger, social media apps are not vital communication tools for young adults. They're just sources of entertainment and distraction. You don't need those real-time updates throughout the day while you're working. Push notifications are interruptions that not only fragment attention and eliminate the centralization of mental resources towards a given task but also provide a foot in the door for use of social media.

Facebook is "a pageantry of vanity," a parade of dream vacations and glossy meals and tight bodies and mind-blowing parties.[46] The design of social media encourages superficial content, which, as we know, makes us vulnerable to comparison, insecurity, and feelings of inferiority. Scrolling through your Facebook news feed and browsing profiles feeds the social anxiety feedback loop. If you can't give it up altogether, set aside a specific amount of time each day that you'll allow yourself to devote to news feed reading and profile browsing. Set a timer. Reward yourself when you stick to your allotted time.

There is nothing on those news feeds or profiles that will make you happier, better informed, or even more connected. They are time wasters, and little more.

A.T.

STEP FIVE: SEPARATE YOURSELF FROM YOUR PHONE

Fearing and simultaneously craving the distraction afforded by social media apps led me to delete almost every single unnecessary app on my phone. This helped improve my productivity. But the most improvement came from physically separating from my phone when I was working. Even after limiting notifications down to text messages, just having my phone within reach was still distracting, keeping my mind in a state of reactivity that prevented me from being able to fully focus. And it turns out that I'm definitely not alone. New research from the University of Texas found that even when a smart phone was turned off, the very fact of having it within reach significantly reduced the cognitive capacity of study participants.[47]

Without my phone at hand I am able to expend much less energy resisting the temptation to pick it up, and I can focus on singular tasks for more sustained periods of time. Stow your phone away and go to the library to do your school work. Or, if you're in the workforce, leave your phone at home. If you can't physically separate yourself from your phone, at the very least, turn it off and put it in your backpack or a drawer of your desk—out of sight, out of mind.

And buy a watch. People often check their phones just to see the time, but they are then sucked into the time warp of notifications and the other endless distractions offered up by that little glowing screen. Just wear a watch. It's easier.

I would also buy an alarm clock instead of relying on your phone. Starting the morning with a slew of noti-

TRAPPED IN THE WEB

fications waiting on your phone? Another way to fall into the vortex. If you use your phone as an alarm, at least leave it on airplane mode.

A.T.

KEY RECOMMENDATION

For better or for worse, social media is now woven into the very fabric of our lives, especially for millennials. We probably can't jettison Facebook and Instagram and Snapchat altogether, but we can make the choice to use social media minimally so that we can maximize happiness and productivity. Infrequently upload content and maintain a basic profile, maximize your visibility for dating and social opportunities among a select group of friends, and use Messenger to connect with friends as needed. Give yourself a specific, limited amount of time to devote to profile and news feed browsing each day if you just can't give it up. Don't exceed it. Use your phone judiciously—as a tool, not as a toy.

Self-control, like any mental faculty, can be developed through proper training and repeated exercise, but if prolonged efforts to establish a healthy, limited relationship with social media all come to naught, it might be time to think about deleting your social media accounts altogether. Here's a question to ask yourself: Is social media an occasional diversion from your actual life, or is it the other way around?

Do you live in the matrix, or in the real world?

TRAPPED IN THE WEB

PART 2: PORN AND RAW YOUTH

Watching too much porn made you feel like you were out in the cold with your nose pressed against a window, watching strangers at a party, wishing you could join them. But the weird thing was, you could join them. All you had to do was open the door and walk inside and everybody would be happy to see you. So why were you still outside, standing on your tiptoes, feeling sorry for yourself?

— Tom Perrotta

A.T.

This isn't a book about pornography—the business, or the people who work in it. I haven't interviewed actors or directors in the industry. I don't know if the actors are paid well or if they have nice lives or if they are happy. I imagine many of them suffer, but I can't know for sure. This is a book about the consequences and effects of ingesting pornography, how it maims people's expectations, damages libidos, and twists our sexual desires into something industrial and pre-packaged. We end up paying for something that was ours to begin with—our fantasies.

Others have written about the pornification of America, where the porn industry has invaded much of our public sphere. A creeping sexualization has seeped into everything from children's cartoons to mainstream commercials. Writing on porn tends to be academic. The larger culture hasn't grappled with porn in any kind of meaningful way. In fact, I would argue that most businesses now see porn and the accoutrements of porn as another tool in the marketing toolbox.

Look: Porn makes tons of money, as much, or more, for giant tech aggregators as for the producers. This is an important fact. Much of the money made in the porn business is flowing to slick tech people who don't have the whiff of disreputability that attaches to people in the adult film industry. These business people operate with impunity, despite making their money off of other people having sex. I'll return to this idea, but we want to keep it in mind.

Pornography is a complex subject. I'm sure there are people who use it and interact with it and watch it in ways that aren't harmful. Who these people are, I don't know, but I imagine they might exist. I've heard talking heads on the news refer to porn using a menagerie of contradictory terms—sexist, feminist, degrading, liberating. I'm going to sidestep the morality of porn. Instead, I want to focus on how porn harms young people who watch it.

Porn shapes young people's understanding of not just sex but also romance, dating, desire, and intimacy. Free, easily accessible pornography is one of the major forces in young people's lives today. Quite recently there has been great academic coverage of the porn problem by Dr. Mary Anne Layden, psychotherapist and Director of Education at the Center for Cognitive Therapy at Penn, Gary Wilson, author of *Your Brain on Porn,* and scientist Simone Kühn at the Max Plank Institute in Germany. Their arguments and findings were essential to my thinking for this book. But unfortunately, considering the magnitude of the consequences, there has not been nearly enough popular discussion of their work. Porn is too ingrained in our society, and not enough people realize how dire its consequences are.

In the 2012 book *Porned Out,* Brian McDougal compares the widespread use of porn today to the widespread use of cigarettes in the past: "It's hard to imagine that a whole generation chain-smoked cigarettes without having any idea how harmful they are, but the same thing is happening today with online pornography."[48]

Young people are entranced, mesmerized, and held captive by the short-term gratification provided by pornography. As my friend said: "It's one thing with cigarettes where everyone knows it's bad, and there's peer pressure to stop doing it, but with porn that's not

A.T.

the case." Another person I interviewed told me: "It's really hard to stop. It's very easy to slip back into it." Without a clear sense of the harm porn is causing them or of why they should quit, young people find it too difficult to avoid the temptation to succumb to easy pleasure.

TRAPPED IN THE WEB

LIKE CRACK, ONLY IT'S FREE

When I was in high school, I experienced symptoms of depression and apathy. I even received antidepressants from a therapist. The cause of my depression? I have no doubt it was partially due to heavy consumption of Internet pornography. At the time, though, it was impossible for me to realize that porn was a culprit. I shielded my relationship with porn from family and friends because even though an estimated 87 percent of college-age men consume pornography, I still felt that pornography was taboo, a dirty secret.[49] I felt I had no one to talk to, no one to help me identify the root cause of my problems. And while I may have subconsciously connected my porn use to my apathy, I denied what I sensed was true in order to continue getting the short-term fix that porn so reliably provided. I was a successful student and a successful athlete. It was easy to turn a blind eye, to gather my short-term highs, and ignore the costs. I was addicted to pornography.

And I wasn't alone. Many young adult males consider themselves "addicted" to porn (one study found that 33 percent of men ages eighteen to thirty think they are or might be addicted[50], up to 65 percent of young men cop to watching porn at least once a week[51]). Women watch porn, too; 18 percent of women reported watching porn at least once a week.[52]

In *Your Brain on Porn*, author Gary Wilson describes addiction: "What all addiction assessments share is 'continued use despite negative consequences.'"[53]

We crave it, we use it, we feel terrible afterwards. Then we want more.

A.T.

And the Internet affords us an infinite, free supply. Ultimately, what separates Internet pornography from its pornographic forebears is what sex researcher Alvin Cooper called the "triple-A engine"—"accessibility, affordability, and anonymity." All the pornographic content you could ever imagine available for free, at the tips of your fingers.

Are you addicted to this enticing medium? If you have difficulty falling asleep without porn you are probably addicted. If you look at porn, or want to look at porn, every day, you're probably addicted.

I interviewed a number of people—professionals and students—about porn use. One interviewee said this: "If you watch it once, it can lead to watching twice, and if you're not cognizant of it happening, it can take up a huge portion of your life, and you can always find yourself just a few clicks away from quick happiness, and it makes it difficult to focus on other things knowing that, with your phone right beside you, you have access to this entire database."

It's never enough. The Internet doesn't scratch any itches or satiate any cravings; it only has the power to create more craving. Artificial stimulation results in a desire for more artificial stimulation. Porn addicts may require an extra layer of artificial stimulation throughout the day in order to combat the perceived dullness of regular, old life on earth, where people are fully clothed and doing things like grocery shopping and taking the bus. As a result, many of us listen to music while working out, walking to class, and studying in the library, and constantly multitask between texts, email, and social media. These artificial layers of stimulation flood our minds with information, which distracts us from the fact that we're not watch porn but also prevents us from clearing space in our heads for work. And outside of work? We can't figure out how to live with any kind of peace or joy. Don't believe me? Look out the window.

Porn: it's cheap, it's easy, and it's everywhere—that reliable triple-A engine effect. Or, as Mary Anne Layden told me, porn is "crack cocaine, instantly accessible, free, available 24/7." Porn is a drug. It alters our body chemistry. It makes us feel good, for a time. When we don't have it, we want it. And when we get it, we're never fully satisfied.

A.T.

POWERLESS AND EXHAUSTED

For years, I felt lost and confused. I consumed massive amounts of porn. It wasn't cute or funny. It wasn't a young man coming of age. It felt like madness, Dionysian madness, only lonely and chilly. I didn't know how to break the feedback loop. It was dependency, a major addiction. I didn't know how to talk about it with my friends or family. I felt worthless, weak, pitiful, corrupt, soiled, and helpless. I was in a kind of prison. I watched myself as a pathetic creature, unable to escape. I had no map.

In *The Great Gatsby*, Fitzgerald writes: "The loneliest moment in someone's life is when they are watching their whole world fall apart, and all they can do is stare blankly."

That was me.

Dependency on pornography will make you feel weak, but it is not actually a matter of strength versus weakness. Some of the smartest students I interviewed couldn't control their use of pornography. They spent inordinate amounts of time watching clips of people in coitus or searching for something new to turn them on. They felt powerless and exhausted. Guilt and shame surrounded them like a cloud—masturbation and pornography were taboo. They don't need judgment; they need help understanding and controlling their dependency on porn.

Pornography is the head of the snake of the bad Internet. Research supports the relationship between use of pornography and computer addiction in general: "A longitudinal study following Internet users has found that accessing pornography online was predictive of compulsive computer use after one year."[55] As a result of desensitization from repeated, acute overstimulation, pornography not only becomes addictive itself, but it inflames other obsessive use of digital media. Our lives seem less real, less important, and less vibrant than short video clips of people fucking. There's an inherent irony in looking for sexual stimulation in other people's sex lives, thereby neglecting your own. One obsessive activity leads to another.

I used to toggle between porn videos, social media sites, email and texts, Twitter, my Facebook news feed, a video game, a new TV show, all with music blaring in my headphones and the echoing sounds of digitized sex rattling around in my skull.

In his 1983 horror movie masterpiece *Videodrome*, David Cronenberg presented a surreal world where a local cable programmer experiences visions of televisions and VCRs as orifices. (Cronenberg being Cronenberg, he has a butthole in the back of a TV.) The new technologies are highly sexualized—for example, a woman gasps as she inserts a tape into the VCR. Cronenberg saw the trend before it was even a trend: we sexualize inanimate objects. We fetishize new technologies. People—and I don't have to back up this claim because you know people like this, too—have developed emotional and sexual relationships with their computers and handheld devices. We are building our sexual fantasies around machines. The chilly glow of the iPhone establishes in our thoughts a subconscious desire to interact with it more and more. If Pavlov were alive he would study arousal patterns around that cobalt illumination.

A.T.

Sever the sexual connective tissue and the Internet becomes less imposing.

IN LOVE WITH PORN

Our relationships with pornography can become addictive because of the release of bonding hormones during orgasm. *New York* magazine reporter Davy Rothbart explains:

> Scientists speculate that a dopamine-oxytocin combo is released in the brain during orgasm, acting as a 'biochemical love potion,' as behavioral therapist Andrea Kuszewski calls it. It's the reason after having sex with someone, you're probably more inclined to form an emotional attachment. But you don't have to actually have sex in order to get those neurotransmitters firing. When you watch porn, 'you're bonding with it,' Kuszewski says. 'And those chemicals make you want to keep coming back to have that feeling.' Which allows men not only to get off on porn but to potentially develop a neurological attachment to it. They can, in essence, date porn.[56]

In the days when I was watching porn, if I just closed my eyes with the light of the laptop screen in front of me late at night, I would end up with an erection. The light itself would trigger the association with arousal. Our screens activate a Pavlovian association with sex, which makes it difficult to use our devices for work and easier to fall into old habits of distracting ourselves or seeking sexual stimulation with social media or porn. As a result of this contamination, one person I interviewed had difficulty working online or near his devices: "I'm at the point where it is hard to watch a movie on my phone because I know could be watching porn," he said. He had sexualized his device to the point of only being able to see it as a machine for sexual satisfaction.

After years of watching porn, my generation has developed a subconscious erotic relationship with our devices. Whenever I had sexual energy that had not been depleted for a day or so, the puppet master that is my mind encouraged me to reach for my laptop or phone whenever I could. The puppet master tempted me to feel it, touch it, and play around with its interface, to ease and tease the path to entering Pornhub or XVideos. Often that foreplay would start with Facebook and Instagram just to "check in," where I would scroll through photos of attractive girls, which would transition nicely to the main event.

Once you kick the porn habit, it's smart to get a new laptop and phone if you can, or at least create a new user and set different background images and screen layouts to reduce the association between your device and porn.

We bond with porn on several levels, I think: we bond with our devices that transmit light and pixels from pornographic websites, we bond to the blue light itself, and we bond to the porn actors. We also become bonded to the form: continuous consumption of new sexual stimulation through a seemingly infinite offering of online pornography. We reinforce this bonding even during real sex, by reproducing fantasies from pornography in order to provide additional sexual stimulation. What's more, all of this bonding with pornography may crowd out our capacity to bond with other humans. Mary Anne Layden explained to me: "The brain releases oxytocin to facilitate bonding, and it is released when women give birth, and during sexual touch, but when we look at pornography that bonding mechanism has been damaged."

Internet porn is a multi-billion dollar industry. We've fetishized our screens, imbued them with sexual power that, frankly, they do not have. We are brain-washing ourselves into thinking that fake sex is real; that our computers provide intimacy; and that watching and doing are somehow the same thing. The more we damage our capacity to bond with other people, the more we will turn to porn—the feedback loop rolls on.

A.T.

A SERIOUS DISTRACTION

Most of the people I interviewed for this book watch porn at least once a day. One senior at Penn hadn't watched porn since his senior year of high school. He maintained a 3.7 GPA at Wharton and landed a job at one of the best consulting firms in the world. He worked out every day and maintained an incredibly active social life, going out several times a week. The key variable that distinguished this person from most of the others I interviewed was that he had entirely eliminated porn from his life. It's an anecdotal data point, but it's one worth noting. One student told me: "The addiction has gotten to the point where not watching porn has become a competitive advantage in the workplace."

There is evidence to suggest a relationship between porn consumption and academic performance. In a study tracking the porn usage of adolescent boys, researchers found "an increased use of Internet pornography decreased boys' academic performance six months later."[57]

One consequence of porn use that may seem trivial compared to a decline in academic or professional performance can actually be a major distraction and potential source of crushing humiliation. One person I interviewed experienced the following nightmare scenario: He stayed after class to talk with his professor about his performance on an exam. He opened up his browser to show the professor his grade on his phone, and a pornographic video from the night before showed up on the screen.

I've suffered plenty of indignities of my own due to

my addiction to porn.

For many years when I was watching porn, I dealt with paranoia during class—fearing that porn I'd forgotten to close the night before would randomly blast from my computer or that some virus from a free porn site would cause the porn to open and play at random, even if I had closed it the night before. This paranoia was painful and distracting, inhibiting my ability to fully engage with class and siphoning off even more energy from productive pursuits.

This might seem like a small thing, but porn consumption has a way of worming into every aspect of your life. Most people who watch lots of porn feel marked by it somehow. In the movie *Don Jon* the titular character, played by Joseph Gordon Levitt, watches so much porn that he has been caught multiple times, to his great shame, but he keeps watching. He can't stop. A low thrum of paranoia and worry saturates Don Jon's life. (If you want to see a movie about porn addiction, *Don Jon* is realistic, funny, and pretty damn good.) That constant background noise—regular porn users know it all too well—exacts a price, on our productivity, our sanity, and our happiness.

A.T.

A GRAY MATTER

The mental slump—a feeling of being dazed or foggy—we can experience after ejaculation while watching porn is not only caused by the depletion of sexual energy, but maybe also a reduction in dopamine receptor sensitivity, which means that life's pleasures just don't seem quite as pleasurable. Dr. Robert Navarra, a well-known couples' therapist, explains the science behind this phenomenon to *Bustle*. When we're watching porn, "The brain's reward pathways are flooded with high levels of dopamine. Over time, the constant dopamine high raises the bar on the level of excitement needed to actually feel pleasure…. the frontal lobes, which are involved in decision making, judgment, and impulse control, experience structural and functional changes. The effect: bad decision making, like browsing porn at work—or seeking increasingly kinky porn content in order to feel that next big dopamine rush."[58] Porn is a consumption vortex. We consume porn videos, and then they consume us with an ever-increasing need for more.

And more really means more. Phil Zimbardo, psychologist and professor at Stanford, points out that men often watch multiple porn videos in one sitting. And, in many cases, "multiple" might be a gross understatement. In a controversial 2012 interview with *Playboy*, John Mayer said, "There have probably been days when I saw 300 vaginas before I got out of bed."[59] With that kind of devotion to volume and novelty, it's no wonder that watching porn often puts us in a state of acute cognitive overstimulation. This practice of consuming, sometimes oscillating between, multiple new videos is how many men engage with pornography today, and it's enabled by improvements in computing power, Internet speed, and limitless access to free pornographic content. The more porn we watch, the more we are overstimulated and desensitized. Over time, more porn—and more novelty—and more and more porn and more and more novelty must be consumed to satisfy the urges that led us to pornography in the first place. And so it should come as no surprise that so many young men feel like they are addicted to porn.

There is another factor at play in that post-porn slump—the reduction in grey matter associated with porn consumption. Though studies have not yet proven causation, there is, at the very least, correlation. A 2014 study done by the Max Planck Institute in Germany suggested, based on brain imaging studies, that use of pornography may reduce grey matter in the brain. Whether porn reduces grey matter or people with less grey matter are more susceptible to porn remains to be seen. (It's likely that both are true!) Grey matter includes regions of the brain involved in muscle control, sensory perception, memory, decision making, and self-control, among other things. This explains why those who watch porn report difficulty engaging in mental operations in a number of ways—doing intellectual work, exercising, and even speaking coherently. After a porn session, how often do we find ourselves on the couch, succumbing to distractions like TV, movies, video games, social media, dating apps, and music when we need, and sometimes even want, to be working?

The good news is that grey matter volumes can be restored. Mindfulness meditation has been found to be associated with more grey matter in certain areas of the brain. Focus on your breathing and nothing else. Clear your mind. Don't judge yourself. Don't worry. Don't rush. Just breathe, letting everything drain out of your mind. I brought up the correlation between meditation and increase in grey matter with one of my interviewees. The response: "That is the key to fixing ADHD! When you're meditating, you're training yourself how to be conscious and control your brain. When you're able to be that mindful, you can be so conscious in the moment; consciousness is huge."

Another means of restoring grey matter volumes is through sleep.[60] In order to get more sleep (and higher quality sleep), it's important to avoid using your computer and electronic devices before bed. Interacting with the blue light from our devices' screens suppresses delta waves.[61] Suppressed delta waves not only challenge our ability to fall asleep but also limit our ability to experience crucial REM sleep. The blue light inhibits our release of melatonin, a natural hormone that regulates sleep and wake cycles.[62] Eliminating digital media before bed allows you to fall asleep faster and have higher quality sleep. Try reading (on paper!) for pleasure before bed. Reading provides a low level of external stimulation that actually relaxes the mind, allowing us to step outside of our own swirl of thoughts. However, reading books related to my career or any work that I am doing tends to set my mind running again, inhibiting sleep, so choose wisely. Usually, reading literature, autobiographies, or other nonfiction that is unrelated to my work helps me detach from the day and then sleep.

There is another prong in the triad of good life

choices that will help you overcome addiction and its effects: exercise. There is abundant research that demonstrates the numerous positive effects of exercise, not only on mood (exercise is a notorious antidepressant), but also on brain function and cognition. Recent research discovered that regular aerobic exercise can stimulate grey matter growth, as well as improve attention and other executive functions like planning and organizing.[63] And, as anyone who has gone for a long run or bike ride can probably attest, aerobic exercise can even help you attain that often elusive state where complex, creative problems can be wrestled with and often resolved.[64] Next time you feel the urge to click over to Pornhub, head out for a jog instead and bask in post-workout endorphins instead of sinking into a post-porn haze.

A.T.

TOO MUCH OF A BAD THING

Porn is dangerous, but the dangers are hidden. They are psychic, moral, and relational. We don't always see them, though. Withdrawal symptoms—and they are real—aren't necessarily physical. Instead, they tend to be cognitive symptoms—murkier and harder to notice. Despite this, the problem is beginning to come into focus. The Utah state legislature recently declared porn a public health crisis.

Mary Anne Layden told me that this growing awareness is a sign that things have really gotten out of hand: "The Internet escalated the problem massively to the degree that the consequences are magnified and we can't ignore them." The processing power of today's computers in tandem with improved wireless connection and a vast amount of free, instantly accessible pornographic content on the Internet allow people to streamline their consumption of porn. People are getting free porn tailored to their desires, anytime and anywhere they wish. The result is immense cognitive overstimulation.

In 2016, at the Bahamas airport after spring break and right before a flight back to the States, a friend of mine told me to wait while he went to the bathroom. Ten minutes later, twenty minutes later, he still hadn't come out. Our flight began to board the plane. Another ten, then twenty minutes went by. After a total of around forty-five minutes he finally emerged from the bathroom, and we rushed to the airplane. He apologized and confided that he had watched porn and masturbated three times while he was in the bathroom. My friends and I laughed about it at the time, but I now see it as a desperate, lonely, sad act, bordering on mental illness. It's psychotic behavior—nearly missing a flight to masturbate frantically in an airport bathroom, as though steeling himself for a few porn-free hours on the plane.

Phil Zimbardo reports that boys watch an average of fifty porn clips each week.[65] Assuming that most men are not ejaculating more than two times a day, this means that men are watching multiple clips—at least three—per masturbation and ejaculation session, exposing them to an unnatural degree of sexual novelty and stimulation. Moreover, many men are rapidly oscillating between multiple videos in one sitting, while also fast forwarding and rewinding according to sexual tastes.

The sexual information overload we subject ourselves to day in and day out exacts a steep toll. Dr. Robert Sapolsky, professor of biology, neuroscience, and neurosurgery at Stanford University, explains: "Unnaturally strong explosions of synthetic experience and sensation and pleasure evoke unnaturally strong degrees of habituation. This has two consequences. As the first, soon we hardly notice anymore the fleeting whispers of pleasure caused by leaves in autumn, or by the lingering glance of the right person, or by the promise of reward that will come after a long, difficult, and worthy task. The other consequence is that, after a while, we even habituate to those artificial deluges of intensity. . . . Our tragedy is that we just become hungrier."[66] The more porn we watch, the more porn we need to get off. Feedback loop.

You can't unsee something. We remember what we see in our cells. Try to forget what Michael Jackson looks

A.T.

like, or President Obama. Our cellular memory is real; it's part of our neural network forever. And we are filling our heads with naked, writhing bodies engaged in mechanical copulation. These are bodies stripped of names, pasts, families, or desires beyond the most primal lusts of the producers and their vast, hungry audience. These are people, but we see them only as objects. Again, all of this comes at a cost. We are wounding our souls and our psyches.

TRAPPED IN THE WEB

A HOUSE BUILT ON SAND

Spending significant amounts of time in a world where people have sex with anyone, anytime, anywhere may encourage the nagging, neurotic fear that your partner is constantly in the market for new sexual partners. The porn trope that women, particularly girlfriends and wives, are sexually out of control and will make immediate, unprovoked advances on strange men I think may cause some people to obsess over their girlfriends and religiously shield them from other men. This does a disservice to men, who suffer fear and anxiety, but it does a bigger disservice to women, who end up with boyfriends and husbands who treat them like a prized possession to be safeguarded—again, an object instead of a person. Pornography notoriously objectifies women, and when young people internalize and adopt this attitude it inhibits the emotional connection we need to form monogamous relationships. Researchers found that undergraduate men who regularly watched pornography used more sexual terms to describe women than their peers who did not watch porn.[67]

Porn objectifies men, too. Porn often shows men as nothing more than a life-support system for their large penises. This might seem like the setup for a joke, but young boys are traumatized by the plethora of giant wangs on display in almost every porn video. Boys associate adulthood, the sexual satisfaction of women, and the ability to be a good lover with outsized genitalia. Most boys don't cart around giant penises, and most men don't, either. Most women aren't cartoonishly curvy, shaved everywhere, and addicted to rough trade. Real bodies are just that: real and gloriously imperfect, but after devoting hours upon hours to gazing at professionally manicured and surgically enhanced objects on a screen, porn viewers often develop unrealistic expectations for real life human bodies. Studies have found that exposure to pornography causes men to rate their female partners as less attractive and to report less satisfaction with their partners' sexual performance.[68]

In the most fundamental way, porn changes what and who we find attractive. In *Your Brain on Porn*, Gary Wilson cites psychiatrist Norman Doidge: "'because plasticity is competitive, the brain maps for new, exciting images increased at the expense of what had previously attracted them.'" Wilson then explains: "If the majority of a teen's masturbation sessions are porn-fueled, then brain maps related to Jessica in algebra may be crowded out."[69] Young adults may miss out on opportunities in the real world.

The point: none of this atavistic focus on artificial bodies does young people any good.

It should come as no surprise, then, that pornography consumption does not promote healthy relationships. An informal survey of lawyers at a 2002 meeting of the American Academy of Matrimonial lawyers found that 56 percent of divorce cases involved one party having an obsessive interest in pornographic websites.[70] It's hard to sustain a monogamous relationship when you've become acclimated to intense and constant novel sexual stimulation. As one person I interviewed told me, "The more I jerked it, the more I needed to find crazier shit—it would escalate to ridiculous shit."

Though porn trains us to believe that more is more,

that we should always be seeking newer and better sexual partners, the reality is that monogamy has a lot more to offer than a rotating cast of bedmates. According to a 2011 study of middle-aged couples, longer relationships were associated with more happiness and sexual satisfaction for men.[71] Porn is most likely not the secret to that long-term happiness. One study found that: "Individuals who never viewed SEM [sexually explicit materials] report higher relationship quality than those who viewed SEM alone." In addition, the study found that those who watched sexually explicit material only with their partners still had higher rates of infidelity than those who never watched porn at all.[72]

We cannot expect young people to have healthy relationships, get married, and/or have children when the chief driver of their sexual selves is the industrialized sex business, where bigger is better and shapely women are always aiming to please. This is the future we're talking about. Do we really want to leave the *future* in the hands of the adult film industry?

A.T.

A DRIVER OF SEXUAL DYSFUNCTION

I won't sugarcoat it—I think it's clear that one reason porn negatively impacts relationship quality is its effect on normal sexual functioning. I'll share a story from my own life to illustrate. One evening at Penn, a friend of mine, a high school senior, reached out and told me that she was considering applying to the engineering school, was coming to Penn for an information session, and wanted to hang out. We hit it off, one thing led to another, and within only a few seconds of her touching my crotch, boom—I ejaculated. It was incredibly embarrassing, and it was only the first of several similar situations.

It took me two years to identify porn as the problem and change my behavior. Before that I tried any and all solutions—delaying masturbation, masturbating right before a date, concealing ejaculation during a sexual encounter and then trying to continue, using numbing condoms—all without addressing the underlying issue. The only solution I found was heavy drinking, and I didn't want to spend the rest of my life having sodden sex. These problems are exacerbated by the fact that porn and any kind of sexual dysfunction tend to be taboo topics, so we are left to suffer alone. A friend said: "Is it a crisis? I don't know, because most guys don't talk about this."

I only began to connect porn to my difficulties in the bedroom when a person I interviewed wouldn't stop talking about a girl he met on Tinder. He had fallen for her, but when they made it to the bedroom, he encountered disaster. Instead of prematurely ejaculating, he found himself unable to get an erection at all. I knew he had a penchant for pornography, and after hearing about his story I began to wonder whether porn could be connected to our issues—his erectile dysfunction, my premature ejaculation. It's normal for men to have occasional difficulty maintaining composure and stamina during sex, but I think porn has exacerbated that difficulty. Thanks to excessive porn use, erectile dysfunction is no longer a primarily age-related issue.[73] Compulsive porn watchers are insufficiently stimulated in real-life sexual interaction. And since pornography consumption may wear down dopamine receptor sensitivity, porn users experience less pleasure from actual sex and actual life, which results in depression and apathy in addition to shitty sex. Unsurprisingly, research has identified a correlation between consumption of porn and depression.[74]

Porn leads us to believe that sex is like dry tinder, capable of being sparked at any time without the need for any preexisting relationship. It convinces us that normal, everyday interactions—going to the doctor, going to the library, standing next to a girl in the elevator, etc.—have the potential to ignite and blaze into an intense sexual experience. Seeing the world through porn-colored glasses, red-hot sex is everywhere, and that sex is impersonal and anonymous, plastic and pretend, and totally divorced from any values or emotions.

This hypersexualization is a terrible and potentially dangerous mindset, and not without consequences. Whenever we are in sexual scenarios, we may automatically invoke pornographic imagery that rapidly overstimulates us and leads to premature ejaculation.

We may feel unworthy from frequent comparison with others through social media and pornography, and then, so badly wanting to feel better about ourselves, we can't resist the temptation to rapidly ejaculate. When we're young, we often fear being caught watching porn, so we train ourselves to masturbate and orgasm quickly. An effort to suppress premature ejaculation by watching as much porn as possible to deplete sexual energy can lead to erectile dysfunction, which is another side effect of porn consumption in its own right. Many young adults I interviewed had prescriptions for Cialis to treat erectile dysfunction.

Marshall McLuhan helps explain this phenomenon: "A new medium is never an addition to an old one, nor does it leave the old one in peace. It never ceases to oppress the older media until it finds new shapes and positions for them."[75] For many young people, porn is turning sex into a relic of a bygone era. One person I interviewed said: "Porn was making me feel underwhelmed with real sex, and I thought: Well, you know, I have to do a sanity check here and take a step back and enjoy sex in and of itself instead of something that closely resembles porn videos." Like me, this person decided to eliminate porn all together. He also sees his choice as a chance to get ahead: "It's a competitive advantage. It frees up time, frees up mental capacity or mental horsepower. It's a sexual competitive advantage for sure, because [with porn] you either have a premature ejaculation issue or dysfunction issue."

The good news—it's possible to resurrect those lost capabilities. Dr. Robert Navarra counsels the recovering porn user: "New neural pathways begin to form and healthy sexual relationships become possible with good communication and positivity between partners. Intimate sex is now possible and replaces the impersonal and fantasized sexual life of the sex addict."[76] By addressing the environmental influence of porn, many young men can eliminate erectile dysfunction and premature ejaculation. Although it is obviously more challenging if your porn habits were established during the formative years of youth and you're still trying to address the problem at age twenty-five when the mind is less malleable, the brain *can* still recalibrate itself. There is hope!

If all of life is sex, as Freud believed, then the stimulation we derive in life is a derivative of sexual stimulation, from the beautiful symmetry and classical features of a building that we associate with charm and elegance to the walk on a beach or in lush areas of nature, where in the past there would have been opportunities for mating. We are sexual creatures, and we have evolved to procreate and extend our genes. But by constantly depleting our sexual energy through non-stop, compulsive masturbation to pornography, we deprive ourselves of that fundamental driver of human existence. We rob ourselves of the ability to enjoy not only sex, but also life itself.

A.T.

BREAKING FREE FROM THE PORN MACHINE

I eliminated porn from my life. I have more sexual energy and sensitivity. And although this doesn't help on the premature ejaculation front, I've managed to mostly eliminate the hypersexualized mindset of pornography. I've also trained myself to last longer in bed by masturbating for longer periods before ejaculation and continuing after an early ejaculation.

Be patient; it takes a while to rid your mind of all the hypersexualized porn imagery. Remember: we store what we see on a cellular level. Exorcising hundreds if not thousands of hours of naked contortions takes time. It takes effort. It takes willpower. At the time of writing, I've been off porn for several months now, and the images still linger, haunting me at the most inopportune moments, but they are much less vivid and appear in my mind's eye much less frequently than they once did. I am hopeful that they will soon disappear altogether. Even after just a few months, all the willpower I've expended and psychic pain I've suffered in the battle against porn has been worth it. Mary Anne Layden says, "By indulging ourselves in porn, we are missing the feast, and the feast is love."

The benefits of quitting porn go far beyond improved sex and relationships. With porn, you can masturbate and ejaculate so often that your body becomes completely weak, drained of energy, and vulnerable to sickness. A phenomenon known as the Coolidge Effect explains how porn makes excessive, exhausting rates of masturbation and ejaculation possible. The Coolidge Effect describes the fact that male (and maybe female) animals can continue mating as long as they are presented with new sexual partners. Internet porn offers an all-you-can-watch buffet of sexual partners. Over the past two years, each of the only two times I have been seriously ill for extended periods of time followed a day of double-masturbation, when I had normally been masturbating once every two or three days. Okay, not scientific, but is there anyone who really believes that epic jacking off—while toggling through video clips—is good for you?

Porn sapped my energy and my resolve. When I was addicted to porn I would have a surge of energy for a short period of time when focusing on a new project, but I couldn't come close to sustaining that energy for the length of time necessary to determine whether or not the business or creative idea was valuable. Instead, I would burn out and move on to the next thing. I didn't have the oomph or grit for follow through.

Who knows what great ideas I let die?

Case made; quit porn; reap the rewards.

And yet, easier said than done.

I first cut back my use of porn to once every four days. While I advocate for a gradual withdrawal from artificial sexual stimulation, lots of people may feel that an abrupt and complete cut-off is actually easier than a slow weaning process. You have to decide what is best for you. For me, complete abstention from porn was too challenging and simply did not last for very long, and then my porn consumption reverted to where it was before—if not worse. But for some people going cold turkey, and even eliminating masturbation entirely for a recommended ninety days, may be the only path. This requires an incredible amount of willpower, which you'll need to bolster and replenish through stress reduction—exercise, meditation, and sleep are all key.

Here was my approach:

Stage one: Reduce porn consumption to one video per sitting.

Stage two: Limit porn viewings (still at one per sitting) to four times a week.

Stage three: Limit porn viewings to twice a week.

Stage four: Eliminate porn visuals. Masturbate only to porn audio.

Stage five: Eliminate porn altogether. Masturbate to photos.

Stage six: Eliminate computer during masturbation. Masturbate to print erotica.

Stage seven: Masturbate only to fantasies. As much as possible, try to conjure fantasies involving real people and real-life scenarios. (Avoid porn imagery while masturbating. Masturbating to pornographic fantasies can restore the pathways that will lead you right back to porn.)

Stage eight: Masturbate without fantasizing at all (this will force you to only masturbate when you truly need to and will dismantle your hypersexualized mindset). This may seem really challenging at first, but it is very liberating and well-worth the struggle.

Stage nine: Reduce frequency of masturbation sessions.

The stages can last as long as you need them to—remain at each stage until you feel ready to move on, but as a general guideline you can aim to spend two weeks at each stage. The main advantage to this gradual withdrawal? Nothing succeeds like success. Each step is only a small change, but you'll feel like a hero when you succeed in making that small change. Then you'll be more motivated to keep going to the next stage. Remember—this won't be an overnight transformation. You are rewiring your brain, withdrawing from a powerful habitual behavior with incredibly addictive short-term benefits. Our minds, seeking to maximize short-term gratification, are not fond of being separated from pornography, which provides instant access to super-stimulation and guaranteed gratification. My mind constantly tempted me to return to porn through random vivid flashbacks and mental recreation of pornographic fantasies throughout the day and in my sleep, which provided a short-term jolt and pull towards porn that I had to spend concerted energy combatting. By reducing the amount of sexual information I consumed—whether digitally (on social media, for example) or in the real world (by sneaking glances at women, for example; I know this sounds a bit creepy, but it's a lot less creepy than binge-watching pornos and beating off multiple times a day)—I was able to reduce these flashbacks.

Keep in mind that the restlessness of having to endure nights without masturbation will subside in time. I noticed that my process of extending the length of time between masturbation sessions has alleviated my restlessness at night. I now only become restless after not masturbating (or having sexual intercourse) for five, six, or seven days, as opposed to the nightly restlessness I suffered before. Life is better.

Be patient and gentle with yourself through this

process. Be proud of yourself for committing to this. It's also a moment to consider what is driving you to seek out porn as an opiate—external stress, isolation, absence of close relationships with friends and family, lack of interests and hobbies? While addressing these underlying forces is important, getting rid of porn is a great place to start. Finding a supportive community can help. When you make a commitment to yourself to eliminate porn, share that commitment with your friends. See if they will commit with you. In the absence of a real-life peer group, or in addition to it, I recommend the NoFap website, where you can be a part of an online support group—read questions asked and answered, success stories, and other comments and ideas from others who are also in the process of eliminating their use of porn. Porn is everywhere in our culture; most young people are grappling with it.

I have to stress—grappling with your porn habit is a *process*. After finally eliminating porn and all forms of digitally aided masturbation (including erotica, audio porn, and Instagram models) from my life and beginning to masturbate only once a week, my dreams were still riddled with intense, vivid flashbacks of highly sexualized porn scenes with myself as the voyeur or cameraman. Your mind will always try to get you back to that place of quick and easy stimulation and satisfaction. You might notice that the real-world fantasies you construct while masturbating will include women with physical qualities that resemble those of porn actresses. It's hard to deny biology, but it's likely that the desire for those hypersexualized qualities is amplified by consumption of porn. Be wary of the mind reigniting the pornified pathways that will lead you right back to porn by tempting you to date women with those same porny, hypersexualized physical qualities. Yes, people may have slightly higher levels of attraction to different body types biologically, but a lot of what we think we find attractive is constructed by our environment and should be pursued with caution for fear of reopening the pornified past.

When I was in porn recovery my mind played other tricks on me, resurrecting symptoms of depression and anxiety in order to inflame external stress and increase the temptation to use porn, bringing back melancholic thoughts that had haunted me in the past to encourage me to use porn to soothe my mind and pave over those uncomfortable feelings. Over time, these thoughts diminished, but they were difficult to deal with and required that I have alternative emotional connections in place to channel those feelings. This is why I chose the summer, when I was home with my family, to initiate this process.

In college we are particularly vulnerable to pornography. Without the external regulation of school and parents and with an abundance of unstructured time, many students struggle to summon the internal regulation necessary to resist heavy porn use. One interviewee puts it this way: "Watching porn is so easy in college—you have your own room and your own space. At home, you have to lock your door and put on your headphones. College gives you the freedom to easily and often watch porn and as a result gives you less of a barrier to entry." Those who can develop and exercise self-control and curtail their porn use will have a tremendous advantage not only academically, but also romantically. If you can eliminate porn use in high school, you'll be that much further ahead of your peers.

For college students, summer break is a great time to withdraw from use of porn—there's no academic work to worry about, you're often back home with family, and there's more opportunity to be outdoors. Employees who want to withdraw from pornography should consider allocating all of their vacation time to a period in the summer, when they can be entirely dedicated to eliminating porn. In his 2015 TED talk, "Everything You Think You Know About Addiction is Wrong," journalist Johann Hari argues that addiction is fueled by the lack of human connection and healthy stimulation. Be with dogs, be with family, be on a beach, be with friends, find a relationship. It will combat the anxiety caused by the sudden absence of the short-term gratification pornography provides, which must be sacrificed to reap the long-term benefits.

I found interaction with friends and family to be very helpful in easing the pain of my withdrawal and combatting feelings of isolation and emotional deprivation. I also recommend other means of alleviating stress: exercising more, spending more time in nature, seeking out real life social interactions, and engaging with your interests and hobbies. These will all help reduce the stress that was leading you to porn in the first place, as well as the stress you'll initially feel as you eliminate porn. They will also help fill all the hours you were previously devoting to scrolling, clicking, and jerking off.

Remember: your worth as a person and the pleasure you take in life are not porn derivatives. Porn is the distraction from those things. Porn is the negation of pleasure.

Withdrawal is hard, and relapse is hard to resist. I was in Charlotte, North Carolina, for a final round interview with Microsoft, staying alone at a hotel in a hellish, lifeless suburban area while still in the process of withdrawing from pornography. Between the anxiety about the upcoming interview and the loneliness and boredom of being alone, I was really feeling the pains of withdrawal. The room was dark, sterile. The walls vibrated. I could hear muffled voices and footsteps through the walls. Everything felt tainted and sexual. I had very dark feelings that were difficult to escape. Were people having sex in the rooms around me? Did it really matter if I watched a little porn? I was desperate to watch porn. I wanted to feel something; I wanted to connect with someone; I wanted sexual release. To make matters worse, fraternity brothers were partying in New York City for our biggest freshmen rush trip of the year. I was missing out on a great time, stuck in nowhere, America.

I resisted. I survived the Charlotte trip without resorting to masturbation and pornography. But it was a close call.

Just remember: you are not alone.

Pornography is ubiquitous. People of all ages, from all walks of life and in all manner of careers suffer from porn addiction, even soldiers. In a 2015 interview, Dr. Andrew Doan of the U.S. Naval Substance Abuse and Recovery Program in San Diego attests to this. He's concerned about online pornography use among the troops. He tells the reporter, "We're talking about young, healthy men that come in here with erectile dysfunction...Young men who can't have intimacy with their spouses.'"[78]

Just as the negative effects of pornography will snowball and consume your whole life, the reverse is also true. The benefits of eschewing porn will begin to compound, creating a cycle of benefits and rewards. After I stopped using porn, I sought to reduce stress by socializing, so I was more confident with girls. I also spent more time outside and became more fit. I spent more time working and did better in school. As a result of all of this positive momentum, I did not feel the need to drink more than one or two drinks on a given night, greatly reducing my alcohol consumption. As self-confidence increases, it becomes easier and easier to resist the urge to watch porn. A 2010 study in Sweden described an association between increasing individual self-confidence and decreasing consumption of sexually explicit material.[79]

A Reddit user describes the magic of the positive feedback loop:

> I completely stopped fapping and viewing pornography....Slowly, I started to talk to girls and become more confident. I felt more confident approaching girls since I couldn't fap, before I would disregard women and say I could just jack off. I stopped feeling so shitty when I finally changed my diet, started exercising, and I also started to go outside more and volunteer, which made me feel really good about myself when I helped other people. The persistent depression and suicidal thoughts started to go away. And I noticed how if I got rejected by girls I didn't really care as much, before I would

obsess over girls and get heartbroken when they wouldn't like me back and say how I hate women. Before approaching girls was super scary, but as my confidence grew and I kept approaching more and more girls, it became natural and easy....When I stopped giving into instant pleasure, I realized the beauty of life and everything it had to offer.[80]

We can break the feedback loop and replace it with something better. I discovered, after breaking free from porn and, later, social media, that I had time on my hands—time to do what I wanted. I decided to fill this time pursuing my interests, my hobbies. Doing this reduced my vulnerability to distraction. I began to attempt more and more demanding tasks, which provided me with real world stimulation and feelings of success, which left me more confident and able to resist artificial stimulation. The result is a positive feedback loop, and baby, when you're in it, it's a marvel.

In a world where distractions and temptations abound, it can feel impossible to focus on your own interests. But we ignore our interests and passions at our peril, creating voids of boredom, restlessness, and dissatisfaction that we will seek to fill with porn and social media, or waste needless energy and cognitive resources combatting the urge to turn to consume porn and use social media. If we don't seek work that interests us and people we genuinely enjoy being around, we risk not getting enough stimulation to resist being destroyed by digital distractions, or, at best, needing to spend an impractical amount of energy resisting these distractions, which renders us incapable of accomplishing anything at all.

A.T.

Choose pursuits that you find compelling in order to maximize productivity and avoid burnout. If you're unable to pursue your passion, look for ways to find enjoyment and interest in whatever you're doing. Being able to identify the beautiful objectivity of truth in math proofs or the elegance of a turn of phrase in a novel can help you commit to work you need to get done, which will help you succeed in school and your professional life. Developing the ability to become interested in things that you may not naturally be interested in is a tremendous advantage and increases the scope of work that you can engage in productively, which can increase your opportunities for success in education and for financial gain in the real world.

TRAPPED IN THE WEB

TWO ROADS DIVERGE

I interviewed someone who had a particularly intense relationship with porn. He understood the relationship. He told me that when he had more confidence in himself, he would have more confidence in his ability to interact with women, and he would use porn less. With more confidence, there is more belief, or "hope" (as he told me), that his social interactions will be smoother and sexual interactions better and thus worth pursuing and saving up energy for instead of depleting energy with porn.

Which came first: the porn or the lack of confidence? A 2009 study found that "adolescents with higher degrees of social interaction and bonding were not as likely to consume sexually explicit material as were their less social peers." The same study found that "greater quantities of pornography consumption were significantly correlated with lower degrees of social integration, specifically related to religion, school, society, and family."[81] We don't know for sure which is the cause and which is the effect—does porn cause a lack of social integration, or is it the other way around? What is clear, though, is that porn will only exacerbate whatever loneliness we bring to it.

Pornography doesn't only erode our self-confidence because it keeps us trapped alone in dark rooms, masturbating the minutes of our lives away, but it also chips away at our self-worth as we engage in subconscious (and sometimes conscious) comparison of our bodies and performance abilities with the bodies and performance abilities on display in pornography. And what's worse is that men and women respond to the diminished confidence that results from comparing themselves to porn stars by reducing their social interaction, which only increases their isolation and attachment to porn. You have to live in the world to be comfortable in it. And no one feels capable or competent when they're comparing their bodies and sexual prowess with porn stars.

Pornography offers us a choice. On one side: a feedback loop between porn and a lack of self-confidence, catapulting young adults downward in a vortex of pornography and deterioration of self-confidence. On the other side: a feedback loop between an abstinence from porn and greater self-confidence, catapulting young adults upwards, with more confidence and less use of porn (and thus less exposure to the associated consequences). Unfortunately, most young adult men are following the first path, like I did for way too long.

TRAPPED IN THE WEB

THE ULTIMATE FEEDBACK LOOP: PORN MEETS SOCIAL MEDIA

Porn and social media do not operate independently. Interaction with one fuels interaction with the other. When we sit alone with our devices, scrolling through arousing photos on social media, we are often beset by sexual anxiety. Then, we turn to porn to alleviate that sexual anxiety on the same digital interface that initially produced the anxiety in the first place. Interacting with porn leaves people feeling chilly, isolated, and alone. Young people turn to social media to combat these feelings. The result? Hamster wheel.

You may not realize that you are using social media continuously throughout the day to consume sexual content and derive sexual stimulation, but often, you are. Track and monitor your behavior on social media by going through your Internet history after you finish using social media; you'll find that you are often scrolling and clicking through sexualized content. If you eliminate porn, you will find that you will use social media less because your masturbation will revert to a normal frequency, so you'll feel less drained and much less drive to social media for a quick arousal fix.

One person I interviewed attested to the feedback loop between social media and porn: "Like X [an undisclosed person] seeing girls he has no shot with in bikini photos on Facebook, where you can almost see what they look like naked, and from there it's not a long distance to jacking off through porn." I call this feedback loop the continuum of digital sexual stimulation, and it is easy to get caught up in it, bouncing from one end of the continuum to the other—from Facebook to porn and back again.

Another interviewee attested a different kind of anxiety that tends to power him through that vicious feedback loop: "There's the time factor from social media—all of a sudden you realized you wasted an hour online, on Facebook—and porn is the most guaranteed, quick, efficient way to feel some kind of happiness for a moment, but when that happiness passes, you're left worse off than when you started." It's a game of ping pong, the way the Internet siphons off your time and your desires. You start here and end up there, only to be batted back to here. You are hit back and forth, spending too much time on social media, then too much time on porn, then back to social media. You are locked in a system, in a game that you never really agreed to play.

Combatting the anxiety of losing time, of being a spectator in your own life, by circumventing sexual interactions with real people through masturbatory porn sessions will just land you right back where you started—everything spent, nothing gained.

Look: we have to see the human race for what it is, a highly evolved species that has plenty of leftover stuff from our evolutionary forebears. We have parts of our brains that are similar to snakes' brains—this is where fear dwells—and parts of our brain that resemble the brain of the chimpanzee. The chimp brain wants stimulation and sugar and satisfaction all the time. In many ways, the chimp brain is our enemy, and the Internet keeps the chimp part of our brains activated and exploding. If we don't try to control this part of ourselves, we are doomed—Aldous Huxley's future-humans, obsessed with drugs and sex and stimulation, but incapable of doing anything worthwhile.

A.T.

ADVOCATES FOR ABSTINENCE

In lives that can often be, to paraphrase Thomas Hobbes, solitary and poor, nasty and brutish, sex can often feel like one of our few consolations. But like any other great thing, taken in excess, sex will exact a toll. No lesser luminaries than Steve Jobs, Kanye West, Isaac Newton, and Sigmund Freud all resisted the temptation to masturbate and ejaculate.[82] Based on the evidence we have, we can assume they abstained with the intention of preserving their energy, creativity, and productivity. While I absolutely don't advocate for a complete withdrawal from sex, I do advocate for a complete withdrawal from the unnecessarily frequent masturbation and ejaculation enabled by pornography. Understanding the perspectives of the towering individuals listed above, along with many others like them who chose to follow a less beaten path (if you'll forgive the crude pun), can help us better understand the possible benefits of preserving sexual energy.

Napoleon Hill, author of the best-selling Think and Grow Rich, took a page from Freud's book when he wrote: "Sex desire is the most powerful of human desires. When driven by this desire, men develop keenness of imagination, courage, will-power, persistence, and creative ability unknown to them at other times.... When harnessed, and redirected along other lines, this motivating force maintains all of its attributes of keenness of imagination, courage, etc., which may be used as powerful creative forces in literature, art, or in any other profession or calling, including, of course, the accumulation of riches."[83]

Sir Isaac Newton is believed to have been celibate for his whole life. Newton sheds light on how he was able to preserve his sexual energy without experiencing the typical costs of sexual anxiety: "The way to chastity is not to struggle with incontinent thoughts but to avert the thoughts by some employment, or by reading, or by meditating on other things."[84]

Again, I am absolutely not advocating for abstinence, but I think we can take a lesson from extreme examples. Why not preserve a fraction of the productivity, the intellectual and creativity energy of someone like Isaac Newton by simply exiting the non-stop masturbation highway?

That energy can be channeled into a whole variety of pursuits. Of boxing legend Muhammad Ali, a professional gambler reportedly said: "There's a kid just come down here named Cassius Clay. If you bet on him every time he fights, you'll be a rich man, 'cause he won't lose a single fight. I believe his thing is sexual control. And he's got it.... Any kid who can control his sex can win the title. I believe it."[85] Apparently, abstinence is no secret in the world of boxing. Manny Pacquiao, eight-division world champion, shares similar beliefs, abstaining from sex for twenty-days leading up to a fight. And like Ali and Tyson, the approach clearly worked well for him. "'We've talked to doctors about it,'" Pacquiao's trainer says, "'Sex lowers your testosterone, so you're not as mean.'"[86] World heavyweight boxing champion David Haye ups the ante:

> I don't ejaculate for six weeks before the fight. No sex, no masturbation, no nothing. It releases too much tension. It releases a lot of minerals and nutrients that

your body needs, and it releases them cheaply. Releasing weakens the knees and your legs. Find a lion that hasn't had some food for a while, and you've got a dangerous cat. So there won't be a drip from me. Even in my sleep—if there are girls all over me in my dream, I say to them, "I've got a fight next week, I can't do anything. I can't do it."[87]

The tech world is not without its adherents. Steve Jobs, notably, decided to eliminate pornographic apps from the Mac App Store. In addition, according to a former girlfriend, he believed in the value of preserving his sexual energy: "Our birth control method up to that point was Steve's coitus interruptus, also called the pull-out method, which for him was about his conserving his energy for work."[88]

It should come as no surprise that artists, writers, and musicians have sought abstinence as a means of focusing creative energy. Renaissance artist Michelangelo was described as having "monk-like chastity."[89] In a 1975 interview with writer and musician Jimmy Saunders, Miles Davis attested to the value of preserving sexual energy:

> Davis: You can't come, then fight or play. You can't do it. When I get ready to come, I come. But I do not come and play.
> Saunders: Explain that in layman's terms.
> Davis: Ask Muhammad Ali. If he comes, he can't fight two minutes. Shit, he couldn't even whup me.
> Saunders: Would you fight Muhammad Ali under those conditions, to prove your point?
> Davis: You're goddam right I'd fight him. But he's got to promise to fuck first. If he ain't going to fuck,

I ain't going to fight. You give up all your energy when you come. I mean, you give up all of it! So, if you're going to fuck before a gig, how are you going to give something when it's time to hit?"[90]

In his autobiography, Davis disparages masturbation: "He [a psychiatrist] asked me did I ever masturbate and I told him, no. He couldn't believe that. He told me that I should do that every day instead of shooting dope. I thought that maybe he should put his own goddamn self in the nuthouse if that's all the motherfucker had to tell me. Masturbating to break a habit? Shit, I thought that motherfucker was crazy."[91]

It's hard to argue with Miles Davis.

Kanye West explains how we can better accomplish our goals by pursuing sex less intensely: "People ask me a lot about my drive. I think it comes from, like, having a sexual addiction at a really young age," he says. "Look at the drive that people have to get sex—to dress like this and get a haircut and be in the club in the freezing cold at 3 a.m., the places they go to pick up a girl. If you can focus the energy into something valuable, put that into work ethic . . ."[92]

Unfortunately, things are less simple now, certainly than when Newton was formulating the laws of gravity and even since Kanye West was very young. Thanks to pornography, sex is always at our fingertips. Virtual-reality pornography, in particular, has opened up an alternative universe that allows people to satisfy endless and infinite sexual urges that they would be unable to satisfy in real life. Rather than being forced to channel excess energy into more productive and creative outlets, it is all too easy to dissipate it with pornography.

A.T.

Let me be clear: sex is awesome. I'm in favor of getting all the hot, healthy, consensual sex you can. Masturbation is great, too, if you can ditch the porn. I include extreme examples of celibacy advocates only to make this point—we all have a finite amount of energy to fuel our waking hours. Porn will drain that energy at a rapid, punishing pace and leave you with nothing left to spend on anything worthwhile... including sex.

We're not supposed to go through life getting whatever we want, whenever we want. "Self-denial is a route to greater pleasure than you can ever obtain by just obeying your desires." A guy named Philocles said that to Horatio in the fifth century BCE. Sounds like wisdom to me.

TRAPPED IN THE WEB

AMERICAN PSYCHOS

Bret Easton Ellis, author of *American Psycho*, began writing stylized and highly sexual novels in the 1980s. In his first novel, *Less than Zero*, the narrator catches a glimpse of a bound woman being gang-raped at a party. And then he walks away. Ellis specializes in this kind of disturbing psychosexual imagery.

American Psycho follows Patrick Bateman, a wealthy stock trader who cannot feel much of anything. He daydreams of mutilation and dismemberment and, perhaps, acts on his fantasies. He tells the people around him what he is thinking, of horrifying violence against women, and everyone assumes he's joking. His psychopathic side isn't well hidden, but no one sees it because no one is paying attention to anyone else. The novel hasn't aged well. (They made a good movie version. If you're going to read an Ellis novel, go with *Less Than Zero*.)

In 2011, the film *Shame* appeared. *Shame* follows another successful businessman in New York, played by Michael Fassbinder. *Shame* is a pretty good movie, lacking all the black humor of *American Psycho* but filmed with a chilly, beautiful glamour. Fassbinder's character is addicted to sex and pornography. He watches porn at home, at work, on his commute if he can. He is caught over and over, but his status and wealth protect him. He is broken. He is a shell of a man. *Shame* captures the alienating loneliness of porn addiction. If a lot of what I'm saying in this book sounds ridiculous to you, watch the movie. Fassbinder is so lonely, it's heartbreaking.

American Psycho the novel is supposed to be

ironic—a comment on the dehumanizing forces in American society, forces that turn people into products and lonely men into killers. It's an indictment of 1980s America, its values, artifacts, and mores. Bateman's most emotive moments, by way of an example, involve rapturous reviews of pop music—such as Huey Lewis and the News.

The key to *American Psycho* is how loveless sex, isolation, and loneliness have deformed Bateman's damaged psyche. Bateman has nothing and no one to help him, care for him, or correct his frightening impulses. He has nothing solid to hold on to. Motivated by greed, the greed he sees on display all around him, Bateman doesn't understand why his financial success isn't giving him happiness.

We are in a much harder, more terrifying world than Bateman's. Pornography has a vile and violent side, and there are loads of young men steeping their brains in it. Imagine Patrick Bateman spending his evenings watching hours and hours of pornography. Every night. For years.

I'm sure some readers will argue that porn consumption might create a way for men to sublimate their violent sexual urges. Through the research I've done, and from my own experiences, I know that porn never satisfies for more than a few moments. I'm not saying that porn creates sickos, but I am arguing that porn augments, stretches, and amplifies unstable dispositions and anti-social, violent impulses.

Back in college, one early Wednesday morning, around five, I heard someone slamming against my door. Bam! Bam! It was another student, hurling his body into the door, a drunk battering ram. He was yelling. "It's prime time! It's prime time, A! Get the fuck up." I had just gone to sleep four hours earlier. He ran around the dorm, before most of us were awake, slamming into doors, screaming, "Prime time! It's prime time!" I could hear him slip and tumble down the staircase, his head thudding against the wood. His screaming resumed just seconds later. I dragged myself out of bed and into the hallway, where others were bleary-eyed and blinking, baffled and furious. We made our way downstairs, where we saw the madman pinned down by a few of our exhausted, angry number who were trying to out-scream him—"We have midterms tomorrow! Shut the fuck up and go to sleep!" He screamed louder, "Kill me! Kill me now!" He was crying, sobbing, yelling incoherently. It was total madness, a psychotic breakdown. As his screams subsided and the rest of the students began to return to their rooms, I tried to talk to this guy. I seemed to be the only one who cared, or maybe the only one who could empathize. At first he was confrontational—"Don't fucking talk to me!"—but then he opened up. "Gone with the wind, my friend, all of it, gone with the wind. My life. Gone with the wind." He trailed off, looked away. I heard him mumble to himself. "Pure terror." Outside, the beginning sunlight emerged.

A few years later, I called him up and asked him what had happened that day. He said it was unhealthy drinking, combined with porn, hook-up culture, the constant multitasking college life demanded of him—everything I'm writing about in this book. He felt overwhelmed, isolated, unloveable, and useless, and he snapped.

A.T.

Porn doesn't just impact the people watching it. As author David Mura writes in *Male Grief: Notes on Pornography and Addiction*, "More than pornography is at stake here. It is the whole fabric of our society, the very structures of our lives."[93] Pornography is inextricable from violence, and it may inculcate violence in those who watch it. Notorious serial killer Ted Bundy, in the final hours before he was executed, attributed his criminal behavior to his escalating relationship with pornography. In an interview, Ted Bundy confessed that his crimes were all motivated, he believed, by his use of pornography, specifically, violent pornography. His words are chilling enough that I think they're worth quoting at length:

> Basically, I was a normal person. I wasn't some guy hanging out in bars, or a bum. I wasn't a pervert in the sense that people look at somebody and say, 'I know there's something wrong with him.' I was a normal person. I had good friends. I led a normal life, except for this one, small but very potent and destructive segment that I kept very secret and close to myself...those of us who have been so influenced by violence in the media, particularly pornographic violence, are not some kind of inherent monsters. We are your sons, and we are your husbands. And we grew up in regular families. And pornography can reach out and snatch a kid out of any house today. It snatched me out of my home twenty, thirty years ago...I'm no social scientist, and I don't pretend to know what John Q. Citizen thinks about this, but I've lived in prison for a long time now, and I've met a lot of men who were motivated to commit violence just like me. And without exception, every one

of them was deeply involved in pornography—without question, without exception—deeply influenced and consumed by an addiction to pornography. The F.B.I.'s own study on serial homicide shows that the most common interest among serial killers is pornography.[94]

And this was all in the pre-Internet era! If this doesn't challenge your beliefs about watching porn, I don't know what will.

As I've said, almost every guy I know watches porn, and not one of them is a killer. Ted Bundy is an extreme example, but he points us to an uncomfortable truth. Pornography is often violent. When we are consuming this violent content, it's hard not to be influenced by it, to have our views of sex distorted, particularly during youth, when our minds are most malleable and we do not have much real world sexual experience. Research attests to the association between young adult use of pornography and sexual aggression: "2016 meta-analysis of pornography research reveals adolescent pornography consumption is significantly associated with stronger gender-stereotypical sexual beliefs, earlier sexual debut, increased casual sex behavior, and increased sexual aggression both as perpetrators and victims."[95]

When we begin watching porn as children, the association of sex with violence becomes deeply entrenched in our minds in a way that is hard to shake, even if we manage to give up porn. And, the younger we are when we begin watching porn, the harder it is to give it up. Of all the people I interviewed, the person most heavily engaged with porn revealed that he started watching porn at the end of fifth grade. Unsurprisingly, he was also the person I interviewed who suffers the most adverse consequences from porn: erectile dysfunction and a perpetual loss of attention span and energy, which he typically overcomes with three large iced coffees a day. One person I interviewed who did manage to stop watching porn was still influenced by porn many years later. After untold viewings of digital female objects (electric pixels) used for sexual pleasure during those crucial formative years, he now has a hard time seeing the value of female friendships or having a monogamous relationship.

For adults, heavy interaction with pornography also leads to skewed perspectives. Researchers found that exposure to massive amounts of pornography fostered a "punitive treatment of rape" in both male and female subjects (measured by recommended prison time for convicted rapists) and increased men's sexual callousness towards women.[96] Putting it more baldly, a 1994 study found that "males who used pornography and experienced more pressure from their peers were disproportionately involved in sexual aggression and date rape."[97] Pornography is even implicated in the lives of victims. One study found that "more frequent exposure to pornographic media" was one of the factors that "significantly correlated with increasingly more severe forms of sexual assault."[98]

As a psychotherapist, Mary Anne Layden has treated victims of sexual violence. She told me: "Not one case did not involve the influence of pornography on perpetrators." Once she realized how dire the consequences of pornography consumption may be, she began to work at promoting research and awareness. In a paper she wrote, Dr. Layden spells out how pornography can become an unfortunate educational tool, teaching and conditioning sexually aggressive behavior in viewers: "We learn better when the learning is rewarded. Imagery which contains role models who are demonstrating sexual behavior, who are rewarded for it, which produces sexual arousal in the viewer, and is followed by an orgasm [in the viewer] can be extremely effective in producing deeply learned beliefs and behaviors."[99]

What's particularly problematic and dehumanizing is that female interaction with pornography may condition not only acceptance, but also an attraction to violent sexual encounters from repeated association between masturbation and sexual pleasure and violent sexual content. This conditioning could explain why more porn consumption among women leads to greater belief in rape myths—misogynistic beliefs that justify sexual assault. Researchers found that female university students' "early exposure to pornography was related to subsequent "rape fantasies" and attitudes supportive of sexual violence against women."[100]

One person I interviewed related this experience: "On my last night with Y [a woman he met on Tinder] she says: 'Do whatever you want to me.' Someone like X [an undisclosed friend of his] and Ted Bundy would have done some absurd and disgusting things." For clarification, he believed X had been heavily conditioned by porn to normalize and desire sexual aggression. And therein lies the problem. Y should be able to act on her sexual desires and fantasies; she should be able to say, "Do whatever you want to me," if that turns her on and be confident that her partner won't assault her or not stop when she says no. But if both Y and her partner have been conditioned by pornography to expect violent sex, her partner might take her invitation to violent, unwanted extremes, and Y might not realize that she can refuse.

Another loop. Another trap. Another vicious circle.

Sexual desire is mysterious. We like what we like and want what we want for a whole host of complex reasons that, often, even we don't understand. I don't want to suggest that people aren't allowed to enjoy rough, and even violent, sex as long as it's fully consensual. What you do in your bedroom is your business, and pleasure takes many forms. However, if a woman has been trained by pornography to believe that she is *supposed* to desire humiliation and violence, it makes it much harder for her to object if that kind of treatment is not, in fact, what she really wants. And if a man has been trained, through constant and repeated exposure to pornography, to think that all women are, maybe even secretly, turned on by violence and coercion, he might be tempted to think that no means yes. There is absolutely no excuse for date rape. We can't change the culture we're surrounded by, where women are portrayed and displayed as sexual objects for men to use and abuse, where male violence—in sports and in war and, of course, in pornography—is glorified and celebrated. We can, however, limit our exposure by eliminating pornography from our lives.

Another person I interviewed reported the following experience with a woman he was dating: "I played the nice and sensitive card with limited success and one night completely changed my approach and criticized her and objectified her and instead of having her accept my advances, she begged for them. It was unbelievable." There are so many factors that could contribute to a woman internalizing the kind of low self-worth that would make her susceptible to criticism and objectification, thinking that she deserves nothing more. Pornography is undoubtedly one of them, and it is one, unlike childhood trauma, for example, that can be easily removed from the equation.

Porn does both women and men a disservice, making them into stereotypes and objects—cardboard cut-outs instead of flesh and blood human beings. In my first meeting with Mary Anne Layden, she spoke about the brutish and barbaric portrayals of men that may condition women to fear them: "Pornography is hate speech against men as sexually out of control and narcissistic and degrading, making it hard for women to trust men." When she told me this, I actually cried. I realized that I had participated in the damaging cycle of porn and engaged with this hate speech during my formative years. I had cultivated a deeply flawed vision of what it meant to be a man. I was twenty-one years old and weeping in front of a stranger. Professor Layden handed me a box of tissues. "Cry when it is so hard to be in an environment where everyone is sleepwalking," she said.

Pornography is also and obviously hate speech against women, who are dehumanized and humiliated, portrayed as nothing more than sexual objects to be used for the pleasure of brutish, dominating men. I've heard of videos of women being slapped, manhandled, humiliated by toilet seats hung around their necks, urinated on. I can't tell you how repulsive and repugnant so much of porn really is. It is a psychosis-inducing

A.T.

machine, a storm of insanity.

TRAPPED IN THE WEB

I HAVEN'T FORGOTTEN DATING APPS

There's a third player in all of this: dating apps and dating websites. Harmless, even helpful, as they may seem, I believe that interaction with dating apps adds more energy to the porn-social media feedback loop. Dating apps commodify human beings, further muddying up the sex/digital self/real life relationship that drives young people into porn addiction in the first place. We are already too attached, in a fetishistic way, to our phones and handheld devices. They provide everything for us, including the possibility of sex and love. Dating apps push this connection into even more uncomfortable territory.

Take Tinder—although I could just as easily talk about Momo, Grindr, Bumble, or Hinge—a dating app that allows users to discard or accept hundreds of men or women in a matter of minutes. You swipe one way to reject, the other to accept. You base your split-second decisions on a photo. There's a bit more to it, but the essential point is this: the app attempts to disrupt and replace old ways of meeting people with this new interface. But the problems with this interface are manifold. They encourage seeing other humans as sex objects; they encourage users to meet as many people as possible, *through the use of the app*; they create new feedback loops, where rejecting and accepting people by swiping their photos feels meaningful in some way, especially if someone you have accepted accepts you back; the act of using the app becomes an end to itself; and the app, as time goes on, tends to not really be about dating at all, just hooking up.

A.T.

Meeting other people and dating isn't easy anyway, but the specter of semi-anonymous, objectified sex is making human connections much harder to come by. And what is one sure-fire way to alleviate all this tension? Drum roll, please—masturbation to pornography! You've got it.

Or, yet another goddamn feedback loop.

Don't you see? Each new thing adds addictive dimensions to the Internet superstructure. Each new element increases the parameters of the feedback loops that so many people are already stuck in.

The prevalence of dating apps is aided and abetted by the hookup culture that has been rampant on campuses for decades. It's hard to say exactly why hookup culture has taken hold, but porn, which trains us to seek novelty and frequency in sex, above all else, is surely one culprit. Social media, which consumes so many of our waking hours, making time to date an impossibility, is another. Sherry Turkle explains: "Research portrays Americans as increasingly insecure, isolated, and lonely . . . Even high school and college students, during seasons of life when time should be most abundant, say that they don't date but 'hook up' because "who has the time?"[101] Twenty years ago, college students hooked up with people they met at parties. Today's time-crunched students often turn to dating apps to find bedfellows. We're too busy to meet people in person, let alone date, because we're spending all of our free moments engaged with digital media, so we turn to dating apps—yet more digital media—to save us. Another feedback loop.

Humans need connection and affection, and hookup culture offers only the most superficial versions of those fundamental needs. Mary Anne Layden told me that hookup culture is damaging for both men and women "because there is hardly any communication and satisfaction." We're not really getting what we want, and we're sure as hell not getting what we need.

Dating apps are powerful tools for interacting with people that you may not otherwise be exposed to, but they are highly addictive and cognitively obsessive because of their multiple layers of variable reward—Whose profile will you be shown next? Which profile will match with you next? When will that profile match with you next? Will your response be positive or negative, and when will you receive your next response? This causes impulsive checking of notifications, tethering users to their phones with a tighter and tighter cord.

In many ways, our experience on dating apps is similar to gambling: we never know when we might win, so we keep playing. The combination of unpredictability and anticipation (variable reward), in tandem with the sexual arousal spurred by those endless waves of alluring photos, make interaction with dating apps a highly stimulating experience, likely causing a significant dopamine release from our brain's reward system. And, as we know, that way lies obsession and addiction. You will never reach a stopping point. There will always be one more swipe.

Dating apps provide a perceived abundance of choice, which has been shown to produce dissatisfaction in the real world. Sherry Turkle writes, "The psychologists David Myers and Robert Lane independently concluded that in American society today, abundance of choice (and this would apply to choices in products, career paths, or people) often leads to depression and feelings of loneliness."[102] Being presented with apparently infinite choices diminishes our confidence that we have made the right choice, and this produces dissatisfaction with whatever choice we make. And what happens when we are dissatisfied and unhappy with our dating and relationship choices, plagued by the nagging suspicion that there might be someone better out there? Yup. Back to Tinder and its gloriously compulsive swiping. Andrew Sullivan writes: "The mania of our online lives reveals this: We keep swiping and swiping because we are never fully satisfied."[103] Feedback loop, again. And the end result: we're alone. "In 1950, less than 10 percent of American households contained only one person. By 2010, nearly 27 percent of households had just one person."[104]

And when, at the end of the day, we find ourselves sad and alone, what do we turn to? Pornography, social media, dating apps, and then back to pornography. The interactions we have through dating apps are costly—they prevent us from thinking clearly about our lives and our needs, and they play into the addictive swirl of Internet activity. Feedback loop, continued.

Communication on dating apps is inefficient because it involves the exchange of what I call poor data. On dating apps, messages can be written and edited, which does not offer the same level of rich connection provided through the synchronous, real-world medium of conversation, where you don't have time to carefully plan out what you are saying, and you can observe non-verbal cues and indicators. With digital conversation, it's impossible to replicate the same level of connection that a real-world conversation offers. On dating apps, as with all digital communication, there are so many opportunities to manufacture and fabricate our responses, which diminishes their perceived value. It's hard to trust the digital selves we view on dating apps, which is why it can take a lot of time-consuming digital conversation to get to a place where we're comfortable transitioning to a real-world date. Meeting and getting a phone number from someone in person may seem insurmountable in a world where we've trained ourselves to hide behind our screens, but it's actually much easier than you think, thanks to the real emotional connection that can be established through face-to-face communication.

Be mindful of how much time and mental energy you're spending on dating apps. Think about what else you could be doing with your time. Think about relationships you could be strengthening or reviving from the dead with the time you are spending trying to gather new ones online. For a while now I've believed that resurrecting dormant connections has a higher return on time and energy than trying to acquire new connections through dating apps. I've also maintained the belief that developing a small, strong group of friends, both men and women, is the best investment to make in terms of maximizing options for romantic relationships. Set-ups from friends can be much more targeted and give much more validation than a swipe on Tinder.

But I'm not totally pessimistic about the basic idea of dating apps, despite everything I've said above. Unlike pornography, dating apps are designed to get us into contact with other human beings, and, unlike pornography, dating apps can serve a genuine, useful function in our lives. You just have to proceed with caution. Recognize that dating apps are obsessive platforms. If you must use them, consider outsourcing to a person who can handle the evaluation (based on specific guidelines you'll provide), messaging (again, you'll have to provide some scripts), and scheduling of dates. This can shield you from addiction to the interface and other negative consequences while allowing you to reap the rewards that dating apps can offer. If outsourcing isn't an option financially or just doesn't appeal to you, there are other ways to limit harm and maximize benefits. Schedule limited blocks of time for interacting with dating apps. Set a timer if you have to; just being aware of how much time you are spending instead of letting those minutes and hours fly by unnoticed is a huge step. Choose your platforms wisely—there are a ton of dating apps out there now, and not all are created equally. Some will offer a reduced time-suck and a much bigger potential return on your investment. Coffee Meets Bagel, for example, presents users with a much more curated selection of potential matches than a service like Tinder, and How About We matches users by the activities they are up for, a great way to get you off your couch and away from your phone.[105] We need to reshape, not eliminate, our interaction with digital media so we can use it to amplify and enhance, not replace, our real-world experiences.

TRAPPED IN THE WEB

YOU ARE MORE THAN THE SEX YOU'RE (NOT) HAVING

Pornography, our artificially high rates of arousal and masturbation, and the culture at large teach us that we, men in particular, should be having a lot of sex. The more the better. And the less sex you have, the less value you have, the less desirable you are, and so on and so on. Particularly in type-A places like Penn where people are not used to failure and are continually told that they will not and should not fail at anything, men and women who develop a metric of self-worth based on sex will intensely pursue success according to this metric. This can even, in extreme cases, cause them to override internal regulation and engage in sexual aggression and rape in order to hook up—yet another link between pornography and violence. By investing your energy in friends, family, real romantic relationships, school, work, and hobbies, you can reduce your reliance on sex as a measure of self worth and develop a strong and confident core self.

It also helps to remember that you are not alone. Multiple anonymous online communities have popped up—people helping each other understand and react to their relationship with porn. I recommend NoFap, the largest online community with 300,000 members, which has very compelling and honest discussions. One NoFap user attests to what he considers a "lifestyle" of resisting temptations for pornography and instant gratification: "I have also come to the conclusion that this is not a 'challenge' but a lifestyle. It's a way of living that says that you refuse instant gratification and instead use that energy towards your goals…The question is—will you step up to the challenge like a self-disciplined man? Or will you bend and sway, snapping like a fucking twig in the midst of a heavy storm? It's your choice."[106]

If you decide to step up to the challenge and my program doesn't work for you? Try something else, or seek professional help, because I cannot stress enough how challenging it can be to conquer a porn addiction. I wish I had tried counseling and a therapist while breaking free from my addiction.

And, finally, build your own support group. Be open and honest with accountability partners. Seek out people who have successfully broken free from their addictions, and receive counseling from them on how they did it. Find out what strategies worked for them, and adapt them for yourself.

Lastly:

Never. Give. Up.

TRAPPED IN THE WEB

PART 3: AND WHO WILL SAVE THE HUMAN RACE?

I dreamed the earth was finished. And the only human being to contemplate the end was Franz Kafka. In heaven, the Titans were fighting to the death. From a wrought-iron bench in Central Park, Kafka was watching the world burn.

— Robert Bolano

TRAPPED IN THE WEB

The Internet isn't just porn sites and social media. These are the two major engines of Internet business and traffic, however, and as such, both fall under the purview of governing agencies. We regulate agriculture, transportation, pharmaceuticals, etc., etc. And let's be clear, the Internet, and especially pornography, is already subject to a ton of regulation and legislation. But maybe it's time to do more.

A.T.

BIG BROTHER?

There are many dystopias. In stark contrast to Huxley's *Brave New World* is the other major work of speculative human disintegration, *1984*. George Orwell wrote it in 1948, following his experiences in the Spanish Civil War and World War II. *1984* takes place in a world where Big Brother—the human embodiment of the totalitarian state—controls everything; every aspect of existence is regulated. The book is read by many high school students, and while it's a great novel, it plants seeds of suspicion and fear that government regulation is a means of controlling the populace, of maintaining a docile citizenry. Yes, we need to always be wary of those in power, always questioning and demanding accountability. However, government regulation serves essential, often life-saving functions—in medicine, in our food and water systems, in manufacturing, workplace safety, transportation—the list goes on and on. Government regulation also has served, at least in theory, to protect us from the most powerful citizens, corporations, and interests and ensure that there are limits, again, at least in theory, on how much power one entity can accumulate—through regulation of the financial industries, telecommunications, media, etc., etc. Let me be clear: governments can and should regulate certain things. The Internet is one of them.

The Internet is still the wild west of information, and lack of planning has allowed a handful of enormous corporations (we used to call these monopolies) to gobble up market share, while allowing pornography to spread its tendrils into the dark and the light like an untreated weed. And if you don't tackle invasive species they can end up crowding out everything else.

And so. We come to the part of the book where I advocate for some basic controls over the Internet and over the multi-billion-dollar porn industry. I don't expect people to like or agree with everything I'm saying. Most people I know consider the unregulated—although I would argue that it's just a *feeling and perception* of freedom—nature of the Internet to be its chief virtue. I think this is a naïve view of business, technology, and society. At its best, government regulation protects our freedoms from predatory interests that would happily buy, sell, or steal them when we are not paying attention. The Internet is not a utopian wonderland of free information exchange. It's a vast, complex business, and it should be regulated like one.

Let's get into it.

A.T.

SUFFER THE CHILDREN

Children have fewer rights than adults, and this is how it should be. Children are forbidden to drink alcohol, smoke cigarettes, drive cars, operate heavy machinery, or see an R-rated movie in the theater. And yet, the Internet and everything on it is wide open to any child with access to an Internet-enabled device. This is crazy.

So, another suggestion: there should be greater enforcement of the minimum legal age for pornography consumption. Even with the legal age of eighteen in place, there is no actual obstacle to children accessing porn—they simply have to click a button that says they are eighteen. The American Academy of Pediatricians reports that "a large survey of American young people revealed that 51% of males and 32% of females claimed to have viewed pornography for the first time before they were 13 years old."[107] This is ridiculous. The age restriction should be heightened and enforced so that younger people, who are the most vulnerable to the negative effects of porn, will be shielded from porn's warped views of sex and violence, men and women.

The strictly enforced legal age to consume alcohol is twenty-one. Under-age drinking is a problem that results in all manner of issues, including not a small number of premature deaths. We regulate alcohol because it is serious, powerful, and harmful. Ditto for tobacco. So why not porn? The consequences of pornography use can be just as dire.

If the proper software can be developed and implemented in order to verify and restrict porn users' ages, we could, at the very least, ensure that porn consumers have fully developed prefrontal cortexes and that they are able to more effectively self-govern their own relationships to porn.

A.T.

PROVIDE CURRICULUMS ON HOW TO HANDLE INTERNET ADDICTIONS

If there is one key objective for elementary, middle, and high schools in today's world, it should be developing an awareness of students' relationships with digital media and technology in general and teaching students how to think about improving that relationship, such that students not only benefit in the present, but also in the future, by not having to spend as much time and energy correcting unhealthy digital relationships down the line. Public schools should develop curriculum on Internet addiction—explaining how unhealthy relationships to digital media develop, the consequences of those relationships, strategies for improving them, and the benefits of maintaining those new, healthy relationships. This curriculum could also cover the importance of engaging in mindfulness meditation, getting adequate sleep, and taking productive breaks from work like going for a walk, reading a book, or heading to the gym. Young adults can and should be armed with the perspective necessary to resist unhealthy digital dependency. They are, for lack of a better word, too young to see the dangers and pitfalls themselves.

It would be helpful to have more science, technology, and society courses offered in colleges and K-12 schools because they will help young adults better understand how our lives are shaped by our relationships with technology. At the very least, if we make sure the regular history curriculum covers technological change over time and how those changes have affected society, history courses can help students understand and interpret the past while also understanding how our society is impacted by and adapting to current, rapid technological innovation. This can help us predict future ramifications of our technology use, be more aware of our own behavior in relationship to technology, and design "antiseptics"—means of alleviating the negative consequences posed from our use of new technologies.

Marshall McLuhan was an advocate of new media education: "Education is ideally civil defense against media fall-out. Yet Western man has had, so far, no education or equipment for meeting any of the new media on their own terms." If you've ever walked down a street or sat in a restaurant, you know that we are suffering a media fall-out—how many people can you spot any given day whose eyes are glued to their phones, who seem to have no relationship to the world, the people around them? Children will grow up to mimic what they see their parents doing—thumbing through Facebook at the playground, scrolling through Instagram in line at the grocery story—only their relationships to the Internet will be even more dire, having never known a world without it. Education is the only way to guide these relationships before it's too late.

A.T.

NO PERSONAL LAPTOP AND CELLPHONE POLICY FOR COMPANIES

Young professionals need help, too. Years of indoctrination have to be destroyed. In the 1700s Samuel Johnson warned of the insidious creep of bad habits: "the chains of habit are too weak to be felt until they are too strong to be broken." We have to help post-college young adults break the chains that bind them to compulsive device and Internet use before it's too late.

A no-phone policy for junior level employees may be valuable. During a summer internship after my sophomore year I was very distracted by my phone. It interrupted my workflow, and my constant phone-checking hurt the overall quality of my work. If company policy had required me to turn in my phone at the beginning of each day, I would have been happier and much more productive. I knew that compulsively checking my phone all the time was childish and damaging, but I couldn't stop myself. Being forced to surrender my phone at the beginning of each day would have helped save me from myself by forcing me to engage in more productive non-digital breaks instead of simply turning to my phone, which was a programmatic but unhealthy response to fatigue or boredom that only left me more drained.

I didn't need my phone for business, and I didn't need it for myself, either. It was hurting me, and it was hurting my job performance. If I need to take a break, I can walk, read, or chat with a coworker. I do not need my phone.

Managers obviously do need their phones for

business development purposes, but they, too, need to be diligent about maximizing the productivity of their phone use, so they should try to schedule their phone activity as much as possible so that they don't fall into excessive, unplanned use, and they should be efficient with the activity that they do engage in. My dad has a great work life balance, and part of that may have been because he is a very efficient digital communicator. I know from experience that he keeps his phone conversations extremely brief but effective, and the same goes for his texting and emails. Although they have scattered grammatical inconsistencies, these conversations are easy for him to write and easy for others read—they get the job done at a minimal cost.

We need to create work cultures that support people in their efforts to separate from unnecessary, compulsive, obsessive use of their digital devices. I think this begins with trying to change the culturally ingrained expectation that we will constantly have our phones with us, that we will respond immediately to every single piece of digital communication. To initiate this, leaders should break the mold.

If the nature of a business is such that employees must carry cell phones at all times to be constantly available for time-sensitive calls, texts, and email, at the very least, all employees could place their cellphones in a basket before the start of important meetings where calls, texts, and email would only be an unwelcome distraction. This same policy could apply during university classes.

Fascistic? Controlling? No and no. We don't have a constitutional right to use our phones. We don't have a constitutional right to use social media *while we*

A.T.

are at work.

Workers' unhealthy digital relationships contribute to significant productivity losses for their employers. Management teams have a responsibility to understand the causes of these unhealthy relationships and respond to them in the most effective possible way. I think employees would be happier if they had a number of scheduled small breaks throughout the day but were advised to not use those breaks to check Facebook or other social media sites.

Companies should allow employees to take a day, or at least a morning or afternoon, each week when they are not required to be glued to their email, constantly replying and reactive. This would allow employees to recover from excessive communication and information overload and give them a concentrated, dedicated time to tackle more challenging, creative tasks without distraction.

Can you imagine a workplace where the bosses tell you not to stay on your computer all morning? Doesn't it sound amazing?

TRAPPED IN THE WEB

SCRAMBLING DEVICES

Internet and cellular-scrambling devices could be installed in certain areas of offices or schools to prevent people from accessing the Internet or using their cellphones. School libraries shouldn't have free WiFi, instead they should be havens from the Internet, places where students can go to get work done without having to constantly resist the temptation to click over to Facebook. Cafeterias should have scramblers, too, and why not? We need to encourage and enable social interaction without distractions. The public sphere is crucial to our democracy, and we are losing it to subjective, digitized worlds.

If the scrambling devices make you nervous, ask yourself why. You can't go fifteen minutes without checking your phone?

A.T.

MORE RESOURCES

I have a few more miscellaneous suggestions, shortcuts around some of the obstacles I tripped over while I was breaking free from social media and porn addiction. Think of the following as a cheat sheet.

Don't read on your laptop. Only one click separates you from distraction. Resisting the urge to click over burns up willpower, which takes a while to build back up again. So? Print out your readings and read on paper to separate yourself from your laptop whenever possible. When you eventually restore a healthy relationship with your devices, you can move back to reading on your devices if you prefer.

Similarly, I recommend reading physical books, magazines, and newspapers. Reading is a great habit, both for you as a worker (I promise you will have competitive advantages over non-readers—you'll have a longer attention span and far greater processing ability) and as a person. Nicholas Carr describes the incredible impact of the printed word on human existence: "The words in books didn't just strengthen people's ability to think abstractly; they enriched people's experience of the physical world, the world outside the book."[109] Read for sustained periods, twenty to thirty minutes at a time, before bed or right after waking up. Reading is one of the few things I know of that has a consistently high return on investment of time, particularly if a book was recommended by someone I know and trust.

Do not fall for clickbait articles. One will always lead to another and so on and so on. Stop getting your news from the web.

In class, take notes by hand. This helps us process material better. Plenty of research backs this up. When taking notes by hand we are unable to transcribe every word a professor says, so instead we have to engage and reflect on the content of a lecture or conversation in order to determine what is most important to note down.

Also, I recommend sitting in the front of the class. It is easier to engage with the teacher or professor and helps you resist the temptation to check your devices. You are watched by the others in the class, too, which provides positive peer pressure.

If you have difficulty reshaping your Internet addictions, even after trying my prescribed approaches, then it may be time to self-impose external regulation. Freedom is a web filtering service that regulates the activity on your laptop and can be set more permanently, whereas other filtering services can simply be shut off immediately with a few clicks. The delay on freedom gives your mind's executive control functions the ability to identify and eliminate the impulse to turn the service off before it actually deactivates.

Or, get the app Moment. This app keeps track of how many minutes you spend on your phone each day, as well as how many times you check it, which forces you to confront the reality of how much time you are losing to your phone. Set a number you're satisfied with both for how much time you want to spend on your phone and how many times you want to check your phone each day—stick to those numbers.

Moment is also an app for analyzing personal activity metadata. With it you can identify patterns and trends in your digital behavior. Once you identify your patterns, you can more easily correct them. For instance, if you discover that, more often than not, you're checking a news app when you're on your phone, it may be worth deleting that news app. Moment allows you to study your own habits. It's fascinating and useful.

If all else fails, get a slower computer. This seems counterintuitive, but think about it. If you require heavy computing power to stream pornography and the like, the slower computer will shield you from some of these distractions. The slower speed and the lag time will help you identify and resist impulses for distraction, which can cause you to engage in less "automatic" task switching and incur fewer associated costs.

The secret benefit of dated machines may explain why the old computers in the University of Pennsylvania's libraries have become very popular. People will walk all the way over to the libraries in the freezing cold to use these older computers despite having their own faster, superior personal laptops. Older phones and laptops (and slower Internet connections, if that's an option) can increase productivity by separating you from impulsive engagement with distractions.

Don't use Facebook as a diary. Don't use Twitter as a journal. Buy a diary or a journal. Write things out longhand and keep them private. Some thoughts are more powerful, and more important, when kept to yourself. Rebuild your interior life. Why does everyone need to know what everyone else is thinking all the time? We don't. Writing helps us process the turbulent worlds both within and without, bit by bit, and can make us more comfortable spending time alone with our thoughts. Writing helps us see ourselves in a clear light. Writing connects us to the larger world.

Go outside. Take a walk. Live and breathe in nature.

Talk to people. In person. Do social things without your phone.

Sleep at least seven hours every night.

Try yoga. Take up jogging or skiing or swimming or hiking. Lift weights. Build muscle mass, stamina, and endurance.

Breathe. Try to be happy. Live.

A.T.

YOU OWE YOURSELF A GOOD FUTURE

After I kicked my porn and social media addictions, I found myself one summer day in a local park in a suburb of Boston. I was alone and without my phone. I took a moment to look around and appreciate my natural surroundings. It was a Saturday afternoon, towards the end of my internship at Nanigans. I was alone save for the occasional jogger, small families with their dogs, and a couple of kids throwing Frisbees. I was surrounded by large trees draped in delicious golden sunlight, and there was a cool wind whispering all around me. I wandered into a small nature preserve attached to the park and found myself standing on a wooden balcony just above a small pond in the middle of the preserve. Bustling dragonflies formed fractal patterns in the air above the water. I looked at my reflection in the pond and took a deep breath. I looked *into* myself. I was growing up, maturing. I had gone through something. I was a changed man.

I felt like I was part of the natural world. Not a visitor or an interloper. I wasn't fidgety or nervous. I didn't want to take a photo of myself, or of the nature preserve, or scribble my epiphany down to post as a blog entry later. I was in nature, and I was a part of nature.

I am a new person.

You can be, too.

You have only distractions to lose and the world to gain. McKinsey, the prestigious consulting firm, puts it this way: "The holy grail, of course, is to retain the benefits of connectivity without letting it distract us too much."[110]

TRAPPED IN THE WEB

Meaning: those who most efficiently manage—rather than eliminate—their relationships with the Internet will be the most successful.

Don't you owe yourself a good future?

A.T.

EPILOGUE

The biggest change I've made in my life, the biggest and the best, was eliminating porn. There was an immediate domino effect. I was a new man. Harmful Internet use decreased across the board. I freed up mental resources. I was able to take challenging courses at Penn. I processed information much more quickly using less energy. My memory was crisper, faster. I came up with creative insights more frequently. I attended social events and didn't feel weird, or awkward, or lonely, or creepy. I could carry on a conversation. I could make people laugh. A stain had been removed from my soul. A ghost had been exorcised. I had an exclusive, monogamous relationship, a big deal these days.

And I wrote this book.

It's been two and half years since I started reflecting, reading, and writing about this topic. It's been a year and a half since I've watched porn or masturbated to any form of digital sexual stimulation. I have not checked social media notifications in over a year. My attention span has increased. I never feel like I'm marking time or wasting my life.

I have a full-time job as a product manager at Overstock. At the office I am energetic, excited, motivated, and ready for challenges. I don't feel overwhelmed or distracted. And because of my new habits, the habits I've created, I not only have more energy, but I use that energy more effectively.

I don't think of myself as very smart. I grew up with learning issues. I never performed that well on standardized tests. I never communicated well. I was able to get into Penn because I was obsessed with a small sport called squash and got very good at it. In the beginning of my college career at Penn, my grades reflected this: I only took three very elementary classes, and I did not do very well.

But by the end of my four years at Penn, after coming up with the ideas in this book and implementing these changes, I was able to take some of the more challenging courses in the school, often skipping prerequisite classes. I did well in those courses while maintaining an active social life and being an active member of a social fraternity. For two semesters, I took six courses—twice as many as I took freshman year. And at the very end, as I was wrapping up my degree during summer session while finishing up this book, I took four courses in two months, including a rigorous course on data science: sentiment analysis and topic modeling. I had transformed from a mediocre student into an unqualified success. And, the key? So simple: I stopped watching porn, I stopped obsessing over social media.

I unplugged. I took the red pill. I exited the matrix.

When I tell people I don't watch porn anymore, most guys are in complete confusion. Some laugh. Some get irritated. Others evade the conversation altogether. I always think of Ralph Waldo Emerson's words: "It is easy in the world to live after the world's opinion; it is easy in solitude to live after our own; but the great man is he who in the midst of the crowd keeps with perfect sweetness the independence of solitude."

I engage in solitude more and read more. I am more thoughtful. I examine my motivations and actions, as well as those of others. I *see* other people. I sense their moods, their struggles. I learn about real things every single day. I am happy living in the world. How many people can really say that?

In cultures where individuals assign greater value to the condition of the community and maintain less of an obsessive focus on the condition of the self, people are happier—like in the Nordic countries, for example. Thinking of others, acting for others—these are signifiers of a healthy person—a person who wants to contribute to something larger.

A way to be happier is to think more about the world around you. Even as self-interested creatures, we have evolved to derive satisfaction from contributing to needs outside of our own because of our dependence on the functioning of other people, and of society at large. But to be part of a community, we have to spend time with other people. We have to invest our precious hours in things that do not exist just for our satisfaction, cravings, and lust. The Internet, for all its marvels, does not, by and large, help build and sustain real communities. Instead, it isolates.

I see a world being deformed by technology. I see people wired into the Internet, trapped in an escalating loop of artificial stimulation. People don't walk anymore, they check their phones. They don't take public transit, they stream media. They don't go on dates, or go to shows, or go out to dinner; they text and swipe and look at gifs and vines and memes.

People, young and old, you have to separate yourself from the artificial reality of the Internet and focus on living in the real. The real world is out there, and it's waiting for you. You don't have to stay in the matrix. You can take the red pill and wake up on the other side.

You owe it to yourself, and to everyone else who calls this planet home, to make these changes.

We have the world to lose, but also the world to gain.

You are the resistance.

A.T.

BIBLIOGRAPHY

[1] Andrew Sullivan, "I Used to Be a Human Being." *New York* magazine, September 18, 2016, http://nymag.com/selectall/2016/09/andrew-sullivan-my-distraction-sickness-and-yours.html.

[2] Hauser, John R. et al. "Website Morphing." MARKETING SCIENCE 28.2 (2009): 202-223. © 2009 INFORMS

[3] Daniel Levitin, *The Organized Mind*, (New York, Dutton, 2014), 220.

[4] Ibid, 337.

[5] Eric W. Owens, Richard J. Behune, Jill C. Manning, and Rory C. Reid, "The Impact of Internet Pornography on Adolescents: A Review of the Research," *Sexual Addiction & Compulsivity: The Journal of Treatment and Prevention* 19, no. 1-2 (2012). https://doi.org/10.1080/10720162.2012.660431.

[6] Ibid.

[7] Norman Doige, "Brain scans of porn addicts: what's wrong with this picture?" *The Guardian* (London, UK), Sep. 26, 2013.

[8] Sherry Turkle, *Reclaiming Conversation: The Power of Talk in a Digital Age*, (New York: Penguin Books, 2015), 55.

[9] Sherry Turkle, *Alone Together: Why We Expect More from Technology and Less from Each Other*, (New York: Basic Books, 2011), 285.

[10] "The Importance of Family Dinners VII." National Center for Addiction and Substance Abuse at Columbia University. New York. September, 2012.

[11] Turkle, *Alone Together*, 227.

[12] "Carnegie Mellon Study Reveals Negative Potential of Heavy Internet Use on Emotional Well Being," School of Computer Science, Carnegie Mellon University, August 31, 1998, http://www.cs.cmu.edu/~./scsnews/aug31-98.html.

[13] Levitin, *The Organized Mind*, 19.

[14] Sullivan, "I Used to Be a Human Being."

[15] "Most-detailed study yet of consumer video viewing suggests some rethinking is in order," Ball State University, March 26, 2009, http://cms.bsu.edu/news/articles/2009/3/mostdetailed-study-yet-of-consumer-video-viewing-suggests-some-rethinking-is-in-order.

[16] Timothy D. Wilson et al. "Just think: The challenges of the disengaged mind." *Science* 345, no. 6192 (2014): 75-77. doi: 10.1126/science.1250830.

[17] Lizette Borelli, "Human Attention Span Shortens To 8 Seconds Due To Digital Technology: 3 Ways To Stay Focused," *Medical Daily*, May 14, 2015. http://www.medicaldaily.com/human-attention-span-shortens-8-seconds-due-digital-technology-3-ways-stay-focused-333474.

[18] Kif Leswing, "The average iPhone is unlocked 80 times per day," *Business Insider*, April 18, 2016. http://www.businessinsider.com/the-average-iphone-is-unlocked-80-times-per-day-2016-4.

[19] Carolyn Gregoire, "You Probably Use Your Smartphone Way More Than You Think," *Huffington Post*, November 2, 2015. https://www.huffingtonpost.com/entry/smartphone-usage-estimates_us_5637687de4b063179912dc96.

[20] Turkle, *Reclaiming Conversation*, 59-60.

[21] Bertrand Russell, *The Conquest of Happiness*, 1930. (New York: Liveright), 2013.

[22] Ibid.

[23] Turkle, *Reclaiming Conversation*, 77.

[24] Marshall McLuhan, *The Medium is the Massage* (New York: Bantam Books, 1967), 8.

[25] Ibid, 147.

[26] Nicholas Carr, *The Shallows: What the Internet is Doing to Our Brains*, (New York: W.W. Norton, 2011).

[27] Ibid, 63.

[28] Jeff Grabmeier, "Multitasking May Hurt Your Performance, But It Makes You Feel Better," The Ohio State University, April 30, 2012, https://news.osu.edu/news/2012/04/30/multitask.

[29] Daniel Levitin, "Why the modern world is bad for your brain." *The Guardian* (London, UK), Jan. 18, 2015.

[30] Ibid.

[31] William Powers, *Hamlet's Blackberry: Building a Good Life in the Digital Age* (New York: Harper Perennial, 2011), 59.

[32] Aaron Taube, "You Lose up to 25 Minutes Every Time You Respond to an Email," *Business Insider*, December 9, 2014, http://www.businessinsider.com/you-lose-up-to-25-minutes-every-time-you-respond-to-an-email-2014-12.

[33] "E-mails 'hurt IQ more than pot," CNN.com, April 22, 2005, http://www.cnn.com/2005/WORLD/europe/04/22/text.iq/.

[34] Amanda Lenhart et al. "Teens and Mobile Phones," Pew Research Center, April 20, 2010, http://www.pewinternet.org/2010/04/20/teens-and-mobile-phones/.

[35] "Social Media, Social Life: How Teens View Their Digital Lives," Common Sense Media, June 26, 2012, https://www.commonsensemedia.org/research/social-media-social-life-how-teens-view-their-digital-lives/key-finding-4%3A-teens-wish-they-could-disconnect-more-often.

[36] Levitin, *The Organized Mind*.

[37] Levitin, "Why the modern world is bad for your brain."

[38] Levitin, *The Organized Mind*.

[39] Tony Schwartz, "Take Back Your Attention," *Harvard Business Review*, February 9, 2011, https://hbr.org/2011/02/take-back-your-attention.html.

[40] "Keep Your Brain Young With Music," John Hopkins Medicine, accessed Feb. 20, 2018. https://www.hopkinsmedicine.org/health/healthy_aging/healthy_mind/keep-your-brain-young-with-music.

[41] Margaret Rock, "A Nation of Kids with Gadgets and ADHD," *Time*, July 8, 2013. http://techland.time.com/2013/07/08/a-nation-of-kids-with-gadgets-and-adhd/.

[42] Borreli, "Human Attention Span Shortens."

[43] Perri Klass, "Fixated by Screens, but Seemingly Nothing Else," *The New York Times*, May 9, 2011. http://www.nytimes.com/2011/05/10/health/views/10klass.html?_r=0).

[44] Marshall McLuhan, *Understanding Media: The Extensions of Man* (Cambridge, MA: MIT Press, 1964), 170.

[45] Shayka and Christakis. "Association of Facebook Use With Compromised Well-Being: A Longitudinal Study." *American Journal of Epidemiology*, Volume 185, Issue 3. 1 February 2017, Pages 203–211, https://doi.org/10.1093/aje/kww189.

[46] Prince Ea. "Can We Auto-Correct Humanity?" *Can We Auto-Correct Humanity?* 2014.

[47] "The mere presence of your phone reduces brainpower, study shows," *ScienceDaily*, June 23, 2017. https://www.sciencedaily.com/releases/2017/06/170623133039.htm.

[48] Brian McDougal, *Porned Out: Erectile dysfunction, depression, and 7 more (selfish) reasons to quit porn* (self-pub., Amazon Digital Services LLC, 2012).

[49] Jason S. Carroll; Laura M. Padilla-Walker; Larry J. Nelson; Chad D. Olson; Carolyn McNamara Barry; Stephanie D. Madsen. "Generation XXX: Pornography Acceptance and Use Among Emerging Adults." *Journal of Adolescent Research*, Volume: 23 Issue: 1. January 2008. http://journals.sagepub.com/doi/abs/10.1177/0743558407306348

[50] Heather Schroering, "The porn problem," *RedEye, Chicago Tribune*, July 14, 2015. http://www.chicagotribune.com/news/redeye-porn-addiction-20150714-story.html.

[51] "Pornography Addiction," UT Dallas Student Counseling Center, accessed February 20, 2018. https://www.utdallas.edu/counseling/pornaddiction/.

[52] Ibid.

[53] Gary Wilson, *Your Brain on Porn: Internet Pornography and the Emerging Science of Addiction* (Kent, UK: Commonwealth Publishing, 2015).

[54] Kirsten Weir, "Is pornography addictive?" *Monitor on Psychology* 45, no. 4 (2014): http://www.apa.org/monitor/2014/04/pornography.aspx.

[55] Simone Kühn and Jürgen Gallinat, "Brain Structure and Functional Connectivity Associated With Pornography Consumption: The Brain on Porn," *JAMA Psychiatry* 71, no. 7 (2014), doi:10.1001/jamapsychiatry.2014.93

[56] Davy Rothbart, "He's Just Not That Into Anyone." *New York* magazine, January 30, 2011, http://nymag.com/nymag/features/70976/.

[57] Ine Beyers, Laura Vandebosch and Steven Eggermont, "Early adolescent Boys' exposure to Internet pornography: Relationships to pubertal timing, sensation seeking, and academic performance," *Journal of Early Adolescence 35*, no. 8 (2015), https://lirias.kuleuven.be/handle/123456789/458526.

[58] Rebecca Paredes, "Here's What Porn Addiction Does to Your Brain—And How to Recover." *Bustle*, April 29, 2016. https://www.bustle.com/articles/153055-heres-what-porn-addiction-does-to-your-brain-and-how-to-recover.

[59] Rob Tannenbaum, "Playboy Interview: John Mayer." *Playboy*, December 1, 2012. http://www.playboy.com/articles/playboy-interview-john-mayer.

[60] Mareen Weber et al, "Habitual 'sleep credit' is associated with greater grey matter volume of the medial prefrontal cortex, higher emotional intelligence and better mental health," *Journal of Sleep Research* 22, no. 5 (2013). doi: 10.1111/jsr.12056

A.T.

[61] Phipps-Nelson J., Redman J. R., Schlangen L. J., Rajaratnam S. M. "Blue light exposure reduces objective measures of sleepiness during prolonged nighttime performance testing." *Chronobiology International.* 2009;26:891–912.

[62] Cajochen C, Frey S, Anders D, Späti J, Bues M, Pross A, et al. "Evening exposure to a light-emitting diodes (LED)-backlit computer screen affects circadian physiology and cognitive performance." J Appl Physiol. 2011;110:1432–8.

[63] Christopher Bergland, "Study: Aerobic Exercise Leads to Remarkable Brain Changes," Psychology Today, November 30, 2016, https://www.psychologytoday.com/blog/the-athletes-way/201611/study-aerobic-exercise-leads-remarkable-brain-changes.

[64] Christopher Bergland, "Aha! Exercise Facilitates the Free Flow of Thought," Psychology Today, March 26, 2016, https://www.psychologytoday.com/blog/the-athletes-way/201603/aha-aerobic-exercise-facilitates-the-free-flow-thought.

[65] "Phil Zimbardo: The Demise of Guys?" TED Summaries, February 28, 2015, https://tedsummaries.com/2015/02/28/philip-zimbardo-the-demise-of-guys/.

[66] Robert M. Sapolsky, "Why Zebras Don't Get Ulcers," (New York: Henry Holt and Company, 2004), 351.

[67] *Report of the APA Task Force on the Sexualization of Girls,* American Psychological Association, Task Force on the Sexualization of Girls, 2007, https://www.apa.org/pi/women/programs/girls/report-full.pdf.

[68] Ibid.

[69] Wilson, *Your Brain on Porn*, 71.

[70] Jill C. Manning, "The Impact of Internet Pornography on Marriage and the Family: A Review of the Research," Submission for the Record, Hearing on Pornography's Impact on Marriage & the Family, Subcommittee on the Constitution, Civil Rights and Property Rights, Committee on Judiciary, United States Senate. Washington, D.C., 2005, 14.

[71] Julia R. Heiman, et al. "Sexual Satisfaction and Relationship Happiness in Midlife and Older Couples in Five Countries," Archives of Sexual Behavior 40, no. 4 (2011), https://doi.org/10.1007/s10508-010-9703-3.

72 Julia R. Heiman, et al. "Sexual Satisfaction and Relationship Happiness in Midlife and Older Couples in Five Countries," Archives of Sexual Behavior 40, no.

4 (2011), https://doi.org/10.1007/s10508-010-9703-3.

[73] Robert Weiss, "All About Porn-Induced Erectile Dysfunction," *Huffington Post*, February 12, 2016, https://www.huffingtonpost.com/robert-weiss/all-about-pornin-duced-ere_b_9220706.html.

[74] Kühn and Gallinat, "Brain Structure and Functional Connectivity Associated With Pornography Consumption."

[75] McLuhan, *Understanding Media*.

[76] Paredes, "Here's What Porn Addiction Does to Your Brain."

[77] nofap.com

[78] Chandra Johnson, "This is your brain online: How technology can affect the brain like drugs," *Deseret News*, January 8, 2015, https://www.deseretnews.com/article/865619157/This-is-your-brain-online-How-technology-can-affect-the-brain-like-drugs.html.

[79] Eric W. Owens, Richard J. Behune, Jill C. Manning, and Rory C. Reid, "The Impact of Internet Pornography on Adolescents: A Review of the Research."

[80] "Haven't masturbated in three years-how my life has changed," Reddit, November 26, 2016, https://www.reddit.com/r/NoFap/comments/5ezyj3/havent_masturbated_in_three_yearshow_my_life_has/.

[81] Owens, et. al, "The Impact of Internet Pornography on Adolescents: A Review of the Research."

[82] http://www.dailymail.co.uk/news/article-2464531/Steve-Jobs-ex-girlfriend-reveals-details-relationship.html#ixzz2i3kKbUAk, http://www.details.com/celebrities-entertainment/cover-stars/200902/hip-hop-artist-kanye-west-talks-fashion-and-music#ixzz2WuqHo76R, http://www.newtonproject.sussex.ac.uk/view/texts/normalized/THEM00061, http://www.wien-vienna.com/freud.php

[83] Napoleon Hill, *Think and Grow Rich*, (New York: Random House, 1960), 155-156.

[84] *Newton's Dark Secrets*, directed by Chris Oxley (2005; PBS), transcript, http://www.pbs.org/wgbh/nova/physics/newton-dark-secrets.html.

[85] Muhammad Ali with Richard Durham, *The Greatest: My Own Story*, (New York: Random House, 1975).

[86] Kevin Cook, "Playboy Profile: Manny Pacquiao," *Playboy*, October 7, 2011, https://www.playboy.com/articles/playboy-profile-manny-pacquiao.

A.T.

[87] Drew Lubega, "David Haye: Fight Night Preparation," AskMen, accessed February 22, 2018. https://uk.askmen.com/sports/business_250/253_david-haye-fight-night-preparation.html.

[88] Chrisann Brennan, *The Bite in the Apple: A Memoir of My Life With Steve Jobs* (New York: St. Martin's Press, 2013), 176.

[89] Anthony Hughes, *Michelangelo* (London: Phaidon Press, 1997), 326.

[90] ed. Paul Maher Jr. and Michael K. Dorr, *Miles on Miles: Interviews and Encounters with Miles Davis* (Chicago: Lawrence Hill Books, 2009), 152.

[91] Miles Davis with Quincy Troupe, *Miles: The Autobiography* (New York: Simon and Schuster Paperbacks, 1989), 171.

[92] Jennifer Cady, "Kanye West: Being a Sex Addict Fueled Success," E!News, February 17, 2009, http://www.eonline.com/news/100270/kanye-west-being-a-sex-addict-fueled-success.

[93] David Mura, *Male Grief: Notes on Pornograpy and Addiction,* (Minneapolis, Milkweed Editions, 1987), 19.

[94] Ted Bundy, Interviewed by James Dobson, January 23, 1989, http://www.dobsonlibrary.com/resource/article/cfeb58f0-967e-4bd5-afbe-7e12206d5ffb

[95] Enough is Enough: Making the Internet Safer for Children and Families, accessed February 23, 2018. http://enough.org/presidential_pledge.

[96] Dolf Zillman and Jennings Bryant, "Effects of Massive Exposure to Pornography," in *Pornography and Sexual Aggression*, eds. Neil M. Malamuth and Edward Donnerstein (New York: Academic Press, Inc., 1984), 133-134.

[97] Leslie Crossman, "Date Rape and Sexual Aggression in College Males: Incidence and the Involvement of Impulsivity, Anger, Hostility, Psychopathology, Peer Influence and Pornography Use" (presentation, Annual Meeting of the Southwest Educational Research Association, San Antonio, TX, January 1994).

[98] Cortney A. Franklin, "The Effect of Victim Attitudes and Behaviors on Sexual Assault Victimization Severity: An Examination of University Women," *Women and Criminal Justice* 20, no. 3, 2010, https://doi.org/10.1080/08974454.2010.490479.

[99] Layden, Mary Anne. "Pornography and Violence: A New Look at Research." 2010. http://www.socialcostsofpornography.com/Layden_Pornography_and_Violence.pdf

[100] Shawn Corne, John Briere, and Lillian M. Esses, "Women's Attitudes and Fantasies About Rape as a Function of Early Exposure to Pornography," *Journal of Interpersonal Violence* 7, no. 4, 1992, https://doi.org/10.1177/088626092007004002.

[101] Turkle, *Alone Together*, 157.

[102] Turkle, *Reclaiming Conversation*, 183.

[103] Andrew Sullivan, "I Used to Be a Human Being."

[104] Stephen Marche, "Is Facebook Making Us Lonely?" *The Atlantic*, May 2012, https://www.theatlantic.com/magazine/archive/2012/05/is-facebook-making-us-lonely/308930/.

[105] "15 Alternative Dating Apps To Tinder," *Esquire*, January 9, 2018, https://www.esquire.com/uk/life/sex-relationships/news/a6170/7-alternatives-dating-apps-to-tinder/.

[106] "The Dopamine Challenge-Are You Tough Enough?" Reddit, November 13, 2016, https://www.reddit.com/r/NoFap/comments/5crla0/the_dopamine_challenge_are_you_tough_enough/.

[107] L. David Perry, "The Impact of Pornography on Children," The American Academy of Pediatricians, June 2016, https://www.acpeds.org/the-college-speaks/position-statements/the-impact-of-pornography-on-children

[108] McLuhan, Understanding Media, 195.

[109] Carr, *Shallows*, 75.

[110] Derek Dean and Caroline Webb, "Recovering from information overload," *McKinsey Quarterly*, January 2011, https://www.mckinsey.com/business-functions/%20organization/our-insights/recovering-from-information-overload.

IF YOU ARE PASSIONATE ABOUT THE TOPIC, PLEASE RECOMMEND TO FRIENDS WHO WILL ALSO BENEFIT.

A.N. TURNER

The author was a product manager intern at Nanigans, a marketing partner of Facebook. Before and after, he spent time under published academic authors at the University of Pennsylvania exploring how our lives are impacted by our relationships with technology.

He then worked at the Overstock.com headquarters as the product manager over the advertising technology team. There, he managed an online advertising system using machine learning models to buy online ads most likely to lead to new purchases, often on sites designed to attract users' attention. While at Overstock, the company's market value multiplied by five, and he learned more about the business context of the Internet.

BEN BEARD

Ben Beard is a writer, editor and librarian. He lives in Chicago with Beth, his wife, and their two daughters. He's written for various websites and newspapers, and is the co-author of *This Day in Civil Rights History*. His newest book, *The South Never Plays Itself*, is an eccentric history of movies, the Deep South, and America, and will appear in late 2019.

Made in the USA
San Bernardino, CA
08 April 2019